MW00469928

Yoga Yājñavalkya

Second Edition

TRANSLATED BY

A. G. MOHAN

with Ganesh Mohan

ISBN-13: 978-981-07-1648-6

Second edition.

Published by Svastha Yoga Pte Ltd.

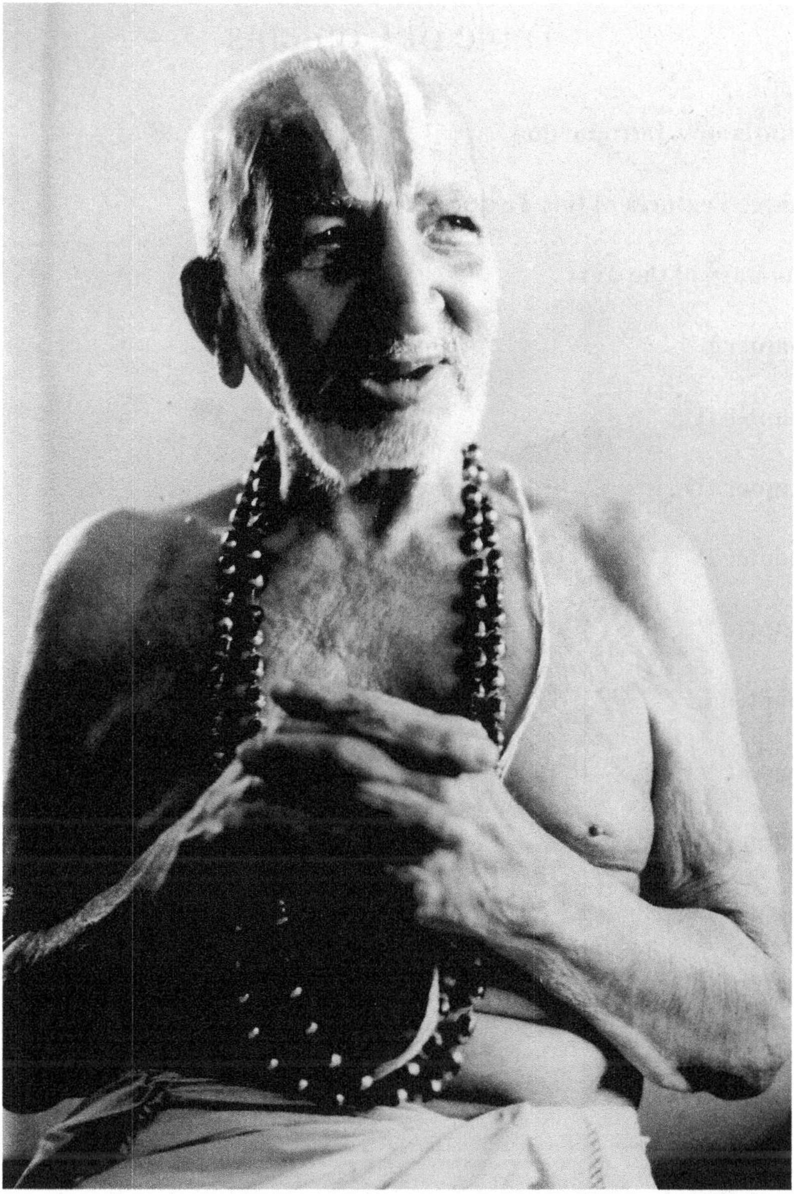

Sri T. Krishnamacharya at 100 years

This book is dedicated to my guru,

Sāṁkhya-yoga-śikhāmaṇi, Mīmāmsa-ratna, Mīmāmsa-tīrtha, Nyāyācārya, Vedānta-vagīśa, Veda-kesari, Yogācārya Sri T. Krishnamacharya.

Table of Contents

Translator's Introduction	**i**
Unique Features of this Text	**v**
Summary of the Text	**vii**
Chapter I	**1**
Chapter II	**15**
Chapter III	**21**
Chapter IV	**28**
Chapter V	**47**
Chapter VI	**53**
Chapter VII	**73**
Chapter VIII	**82**
Chapter IX	**92**
Chapter X	**101**
Chapter XI	**107**
Chapter XII	**113**
Appendix I: Comparisons of Versions	**123**
Appendix II: Devanagari Text	**124**

Translator's Introduction

Recognizing the Yoga Yājñavalkya

My teacher, the great yogi Sri T. Krishnamacharya, considered the Yoga Yājñavalkya to be one of the most important yoga texts. It was perhaps only Krishnamacharya who recognized the uniqueness and importance of this valuable text, as it is little known in other yoga schools.

He has mentioned the Yoga Yājñavalkya in his introduction to the Yoga Makaranda, Part 1 in 1934. He had copied the verses of the text into his diaries from manuscripts. Subsequently, there was also a printed edition from Trivandrum (Trivandrum Sanskrit Series No. CXXXIV, 1938) and one from the BBRA (Bombay Branch Royal Asiatic Society, Monograph 3, 1954).

Studying the Text with Krishnamacharya

My lessons on the Yoga Yājñavalkya with Krishnamacharya began on 25 September 1975. This was not a text that Krishnamacharya considered necessary for students to memorize. In fact, he had himself not committed it to memory. So, referring to a version he had written down in his diaries, he started dictating the text to me.

For some extraneous reasons, the classes on the Yoga Yājñavalkya were interrupted for a while. Over the next two years or so, I completed studying the Haṭhayogapradīpikā, and one round of studies on the Yogasūtra and Sāṁkhya-kārikā, with Krishnamacharya.

Meanwhile, as writing all the verses of the Yoga Yājñavalkya was relatively time consuming, I was looking for a printed version of the text and located the edition printed by BBRA. I ordered the book and received the copies.

When I showed Krishnamacharya the newly acquired BBRA edition, he said that it was more complete and accurate than the version in his possession at that time. Consequently, he recommended the use of the

BBRA edition for my studies. This translation of the Yoga Yājñavalkya you are reading now is based on the BBRA edition.

When I resumed the study of the Yoga Yājñavalkya in personal classes with Krishnamacharya, I had already studied other classical yoga texts. Therefore, he suggested a topic based approach, collating the views of the different classical yoga texts, as the comparisons were valuable and illuminating. In the 1980s, when we were going through the Gheraṇḍa Samhitā, he again compared all the three texts—Haṭhayogapradīpikā, Gheraṇḍa Samhitā, and the Yoga Yājñavalkya—in greater depth, particularly on the topic of kunḍalinī related practices.

Importance of the Yoga Yājñavalkya from Krishnamacharya's Teachings

Krishnamacharya valued the Yoga Yājñavalkya for its systematic and detailed description of the kunḍalinī and related concepts—clearer than more well-known texts like the Haṭhayogapradīpikā, Gheraṇḍa Samhitā, and other later Yoga Upaniṣads. The Yoga Yājñavalkya explains kunḍalinī arousal through pranayama practice principally, which Krishnamacharya considered the sound approach. In contrast, the Haṭhayogapradīpikā and Gheraṇḍa Samhitā contains kriyas and some unsound practices for śakti-cālana to raise the kunḍalinī.

Krishnamacharya was the extraordinarily rare yogi who had practiced both—the techniques of kriyas like nauli from the Haṭhayogapradīpikā, as well as the methods of the Yoga Yājñavalkya. He had written an essay in his diary, titled "What Kunḍalinī is and Kunḍalinī Arousal."

In my classes with him, he did compare the kunḍalinī arousal practices from both, with instructions and practice suggestions. He explained the relation between the two, as well as their differences, and why one should choose one over the other—not just from the texts, but from his own experience. That was why, perhaps, he was the only yogi to realize the importance of the Yoga Yājñavalkya in the last century.

Additionally, Krishnamacharya would emphasize that the Yoga Yājñavalkya is the source many other later yoga texts draw from—this adds weight to the views in it.

Finally, Krishnamacharya appreciated that the text makes clear the therapeutic value of the practice of yoga. The therapeutic applications of yoga were, of course, a specialty of Krishnamacharya's teachings.

Other Translation of the Yoga Yājñavalkya

The only other English translation of the Yoga Yājñavalkya has been released by the Krishnamacharya Yoga Mandiram (KYM). The publisher's note and translator's introduction, together with the rear cover, create the impression that Krishnamacharya dictated the Yoga Yājñavalkya from memory, and that he had corrected and completed the text to produce a version superior to existing publications, which was then passed on to his family, and offered as the book from KYM.

However, a comparative reading shows that the KYM edition is a faithful reproduction of the 1938 Trivandrum publication. The only edits made are to fill in a negligible number of missing words—around 60 words out of 6000—in mostly obvious contexts. There are no significant corrections to existing verses.

The BBRA publication is easily more complete and error free, containing copious footnotes comparing different versions of the text from sixteen manuscripts and five printed editions (including the Trivandrum publication). That is why Krishnamacharya recommended the BBRA publication when he browsed through it.

The Trivandrum publication offered by the KYM misses 39½ verses that appear in the BBRA publication, and the word choice is less suitable in places. Appendix I contains a comparison between the two publications.

About the Second Edition of this Translation

I first translated the Yoga Yājñavalkya more than ten years ago. This is the second edition of the translation. This edition has been revised from beginning to end by my son, Ganesh Mohan. Now the translation is accompanied by the roman transliteration instead of the Devanagari verses, as the former is accessible to more readers. The Devanagari text is also included, in Appendix II.

Sentence constructions have been clarified, and word choices scrutinized to improve comprehension and readability. Some content in the first edition has been removed.

We have tried to stay faithful to the exact words of the original text, but this is a translation from the view of a yoga practitioner and teacher, not an academic scholar. Where exactness would result in obscure translations, we have chosen to use words that serve clarity instead of remaining literal. Some Sanskrit words are explained in English but repeated in Sanskrit, as there is no accurate English equivalent for them (kuṇḍalinī, prāṇa, nāḍī, for example). Still, this text requires much explanation and wide knowledge to truly understand the concepts, practices, and experiences described.

I hope this wonderful text will reach more serious yoga seekers.

I place this work at the feet of my ācārya, Sri T. Krishnamacharya.

A. G. Mohan

Unique Features of this Text

1. The Yoga Yājñavalkya is an ancient text. Many well-known yoga texts of later times, such as the Haṭhayogapradīpikā of Svātmārāma, the Yoga Kuṇḍalinī and Yoga Tattva Upaniṣads, and so on, paraphrase or quote the Yoga Yājñavalkya, or make repeated references to the views of the sage Yājñavalkya. Clearly, the Yoga Yājñavalkya preceded these texts, and has also been the source or the inspiration for many concepts and practices.

2. The text takes the form of a conversation between a husband and wife. Yājñavalkya explains the principles and practice of yoga, the path to freedom, to Gārgī, his wife.

3. The Haṭhayogapradīpikā (II.37) mentions that yogis like Yājñavalkya have a different perspective and do not approve the practice of the kriyās. The Yoga Yājñavalkya presents that perspective. Yājñavalkya describes how the kuṇḍalinī arousal may be achieved principally through pranayama, without need of kriyās, and without some of the more problematic practices described in other texts. The Yoga Yājñavalkya is more in line with Vedic thinking, since kuṇḍalinī finds no reference in the Vedas or the Yogasūtra. Kuṇḍalinī is spoken of in later yoga texts (a fact Krishnamacharya referred to in classes on that topic across the years).

4. The limbs of yoga are presented in a coherent and orderly manner, each in a separate chapter.

5. The concept of prāṇa, its divisions and their functions, are explained clearly, as are the origin, function, position and the connections between the primary nāḍīs.

6. Up to a hundred verses are devoted to techniques, applications, and results of prāṇāyāma. The text also mentions the use of prāṇāyāma as a therapeutic tool, its relation to Ayurveda, and methods to incorporate prāṇāyāma with pratyāhāra, dhāraṇā, and the other limbs of yoga.

7. This book provides insight into various forms of meditation practiced during the Vedic period. It addresses the issue of how we can use meditation on the Divine with form to go beyond form.

Summary of the Text

Chapter I

The text begins with a description of the qualities of Yājñavalkya and his wife Gārgī, who live in a hermitage with many other great sages. In an assembly of such sages, Gārgī requests Yājñavalkya to teach her the essence of yoga. Yājñavalkya consents with happiness. He meditates on the Divine, and begins his discourse.

He describes how he approached Brahma (the Creator) to learn the highest truth—the way to freedom. Brahma graciously explains to him the means to freedom. He says that doing one's duties, with clarity of intention and without desire, is the path to freedom. Doing the same actions, but with desire is sure to lead one to further bondage. Then Brahma goes on to describe the manner in which one should lead one's life according to the varṇāśramadharma. Concluding with this, Brahma himself recedes into the state of yoga.

Gārgī hears this exposition of the means to freedom as said by Brahma to Yājñavalkya, and then requests Yājñavalkya to elaborate upon it further. Yājñavalkya now explains the yoga that one should practice, along with the actions prescribed by the varṇāśramadharma, to attain freedom.

He defines yoga as the union of the jīvātmā (individual or self) and the parāmatmā (Divine). This yoga has eight limbs—yama, niyama, āsana, prāṇāyāma, pratyāhāra, dhāraṇā, dhyāna, and samādhi. Then Yājñavalkya lists the number of types of practices under each limb, and explains in detail the first limb, yama. The ten yamas—ahimsā, satya, asteya, brahmacarya, dayā, ārjava, kṣamā, dhṛti, mitāhāra, and śauca—are then explained in detail. This concludes the first chapter.

Chapter II

The second chapter deals with the niyamas, the second limb of aṣṭāṅga yoga. The ten niyamas are tapas, santoṣa, āstikya, dāna, īśvarapūjana, siddhāntaśravaṇa, hrī, mati, japa, and vrata. Yājñavalkya lists the ten niyamas, and then defines each one of them. He then explains the various grades of recitation of mantra (japa).

Chapter III

Yājñavalkya describes selected (mainly seated) āsanas in this chapter. He begins with a list of eight āsanas: svastikāsana, gomukhāsana, padmāsana, vīrāsana, simhāsana, bhadrāsana, muktāsana and mayūrāsana. He then describes these āsanas in the above order. He offers two variations of svastikāsana and muktāsana alone. Then he says that all diseases are destroyed by the practice of āsanas along with yama and niyama. He concludes the chapter instructing Gārgī to practice prāṇāyāma, along with yama, niyama and āsana, after purifying the nāḍīs.

Chapter IV

This chapter begins with Gārgī requesting Yājñavalkya to explain in detail the method of purification of the nāḍīs, along with the position, origin, and termination of each, as well as the position, function, and movement of each of the vāyus.

Yājñavalkya begins with the concept of scattering of prāṇa and then emphasizes the importance of centering the prāṇa. Then the shape and position of the center of the body (dehamadhya), and the kandasthāna in humans, animals and birds are given in order. Then follows a description of the abode of the jīva (self)—the cakra at the navel (nābhicakra), the kuṇḍalinī, and their respective positions in the body. Then the awakening of the kuṇḍalinī and the upward movement of the prāṇa are described.

Next, Yājñavalkya speaks of the nāḍīs. He lists the fourteen important nāḍīs, and describes the suṣumnā nāḍī as the most important one. Then he describes the iḍā and piṅgalā nāḍīs, and the relative position of the remaining eleven nāḍīs. He gives further details on the origin and termination of each of the nāḍīs.

Yājñavalkya then lists the ten vāyus and their functions. He describes the position of the most important vāyu in the body, the prāṇa vāyu, then describes the location of the apāna vāyu, the other three important vāyus (vyāna, udāna and samāna vāyus), as well as the remaining five vāyus. Then he discusses the role of prāṇa vāyu in the digestion and assimilation of food. Finally, he describes the principal function of each of the ten vāyus. He concludes by instructing Gārgī to perform nāḍīśodhana prāṇāyāma in the prescribed manner, after having understood everything explained so far.

Chapter V

In this chapter, Yājñavalkya discusses the preparations and practice of purifying the nāḍīs (nāḍīśodana). He first describes the qualities that an ideal aspirant should possess before attempting to purify the nāḍīs. Then the ideal environment and daily routine for the practice are described. Following this, he describes an alternative opinion, proposed by some other great sages.

The preparations for the practice of nāḍīśodana, the technique of the practice, and the daily routine and duration of the practice, in accordance with this alternate opinion, are given in detail. Yājñavalkya concludes the chapter describing the results of such a practice.

Chapter VI

This chapter discusses various types of prāṇāyāma, the procedures of practicing them and their benefits. Yājñavalkya begins by defining prāṇāyāma as balancing prāṇa and apāna. He relates the three components of prāṇāyāma (inhalation, holding, and exhalation) to the three syllables of OM. He proposes two procedures of prāṇāyāma, involving different ratios of inhalation, holding, and exhalation. The first three divisions of society may use the Gāyatrī mantra or the praṇava (OM), while the fourth division and women should use other mantras, such as namaḥ.

Then three grades of prāṇāyāma are described. Yājñavalkya explains that the type of prāṇāyāma that leads to lightness of the body and absorption of the mind is the best one. He then explains the concept and practice of kevala kumbhaka and sahita kumbhaka.

Then we are given another definition of prāṇāyāma: prāṇāyāma means retaining the prāṇa within the body. Yājñavalkya explains two ways to master the prāṇa: one using the ṣaṇmukhī mudrā, and the other, an alternative involving āsana and praṇava. He also describes the results of focusing the prāṇa at various places in the body, and how diseases are destroyed by such a practice pointing toward the therapeutic applications of prāṇāyāma. Yājñavalkya also notes the mantras to be used by the four divisions of society during prāṇāyāma practice.

He then describes the movement of the prāṇa to the crown of the head (brahmarandhra) and the sound (nāda) that arises during the upward movement of the prāṇa. The role of prāṇāyāma in the destruction of the kuṇḍalinī and the removal of ignorance (avidyā) is also described. The chapter concludes by stressing the importance of the practice of prāṇāyāma and daily rituals (nityakarma) to achieve the union of the self with the Divine.

Chapter VII

The first four limbs of yoga were described in the preceding six chapters. Here, Yājñavalkya begins explanation of pratyāhāra, the fifth limb of yoga. Five different forms of pratyāhāra are suggested.

The fourth and perhaps most important form is defined as, "Having drawn the prāṇa from point to point, holding it in the eighteen vital points (marmasthānas)." These eighteen vital points are then listed and the distance between each of them is given in order. Following this, the method of drawing and focusing the prāṇa in each of these points is explained in detail, and then the benefits of such a practice are also discussed.

Finally, Yājñavalkya explains the fifth form of pratyāhāra, and how one can reach freedom by focusing the prāṇa in certain vital points.

Chapter VIII

Yājñavalkya explains the five types of mental focus (dhāraṇā) in this chapter. Dhāraṇā is defined as the absorption of the mind in the self. The five types of dhāraṇā are distinguished by their focus on the five deities in the region of the corresponding form of matter in the body.

The region of each of the forms of matter in the body is described, and then, the procedure, duration, and results of dhāraṇā on each of the deities in the appropriate region of the body are discussed. Then the process of involution, which is the objective of the practice of dhāraṇā using the above deities, is explained. Then follows another method to bring about this involution through the use of the praṇava.

Yājñavalkya says that, for those absorbed in yoga, the three doṣas can be balanced by the practice of prāṇāyāma with dhāraṇā. He states that all the diseases caused by the imbalance of the doṣas are removed by the practice of dhāraṇā.

Finally, he concludes the chapter by again emphasizing the importance of the practice of one's daily duties (in accordance with the Vedas) and the previous limbs of yama, niyama etc.

Chapter IX

In this chapter, Yājñavalkya describes the various methods of dhyāna. Dhyāna is the cause for the bondage or freedom of all beings. Dhyāna is to realize the self using the mind. It is of two types: with attributes (saguṇa), and without attributes (nirguṇa). Then various forms of dhyāna (both with and without attributes) are described by Yājñavalkya. The benefits of dhyāna are said to be such that one who does dhyāna as suggested can attain freedom in one year. Then Yājñavalkya instructs Gārgī to do her duties in accordance with the Vedas, and to do dhyāna always. He concludes emphasizing that all great seers have attained freedom through dhyāna.

Chapter X

Yājñavalkya speaks about samādhi in this chapter. Samādhi is the state of union of the self and the Divine. Whatever one does dhyāna upon, one attains samādhi or oneness with that. Surrendering to an entity also leads to samādhi with that deity. The prerequisites for the attainment of samādhi are described.

Following this is a detailed description of the process by which a yogi gives up his body at the time of death and attains freedom. One must leave the body thinking of that on which one has focused during the practice of yoga, because one becomes what one thinks of at the time of death. Yājñavalkya again emphasizes that freedom is assured for one who follows the actions laid down in the Vedas without desire.

Finally, Yājñavalkya concludes the chapter saying that the path of karmayogasamuccaya—a combination of action (karma) and yoga (jñāna) has now been expounded by him and again advises Gārgī to reach freedom by the practice of yoga.

Chapter XI

This chapter begins with Gārgī asking Yājñavalkya to explain how a person in a state of yoga (samādhi) will perform the actions prescribed in the Vedas, and if he cannot do it, what is the (prāyaścitta) purification he must undertake.

Yājñavalkya replies that one in a state of yoga (samādhi) need not do any of the Vedic duties. But when one comes out of samādhi, when the self is not united with the Divine, one must perform all the Vedic duties. If a yogi does not perform these duties, with the attitude that they are unpleasant or difficult, he will suffer for no living being can remain without performing any actions.

Yājñavalkya then instructs Gārgī to perform all her Vedic duties and attain freedom through the practice of yoga. Then he requests all the sages present there to return to their respective hermitages. All the sages return to their hermitages after honoring and worshipping Yājñavalkya. After they have all left, Gārgī again asks Yājñavalkya to explain the path of yoga in a brief manner. Yājñavalkya benevolently accedes to her request.

Chapter XII

This chapter contains the a summary of key parts of this text; Yājñavalkya describes the yogic path to freedom concisely. The progression towards freedom outlined here can be divided into a series of seven orderly stages:

1st stage: Checking the downward flow of apāna (prāṇa) and directing it towards the fire, thereby fanning its flames and vitalizing it. The benefits, or signs of progress due to this practice, are detailed.

2nd stage: The burning of the kuṇḍalinī (avidyā) by the flames of the fire, leading to its awakening. When the kuṇḍalinī is awakened, the nāḍīs are uncovered and the prāṇa begins to flow in the suṣumnā.

3rd stage: Movement of the prāṇa and the fire upwards to the heart-lotus through the suṣumnā and the awakening or blooming of the heart-lotus. The manifestation of various signs, internal and external, as a result of this practice.

4th stage: Further upward movement of the prāṇa, meditation using praṇava and visualization of the disc of the moon in the forehead.

5th stage: The concentration of the prāṇa, and the absorption of the mind, with meditation on the inner self, between the eyebrows, enabling one to see in oneself an effulgent liṅga. Various signs like a trembling in the head, appearance of visions of celestial gardens, the moon, the stars etc. indicate one's progress.

6th stage: Meditation on the Divine (Viṣṇu) in his abode, in the middle of the eyebrows. This is a state said to be very close to the attainment of freedom.

7th stage: The attainment of freedom, and the splitting of the crown of the head, following the advice of one's guru.

Yājñavalkya reiterates the benefits of yoga practice, and concludes his discourse, again emphasizing the importance of the practice of one's daily duties according to the Vedas. Then Yājñavalkya recedes into samādhi in solitude and Gārgī, having understood the essence of yoga, worships Yājñavalkya and does the same.

The text concludes with a verse in praise of Vāsudeva (the Divine) and a verse to the effect that Yājñavalkya and Gārgī are always present, seeing the Divine within themselves.

Chapter I

OUTLINE

1-5: The qualities of sage Yājñavalkya.

6-8: Gārgī's request to Yājñavalkya to teach her the essence of yoga.

9-19: Yājñavalkya meditates on the Divine (in the form of Nārāyaṇa) and describes how he approached the Creator (Brahma), to learn the highest truth.

19-27: The path to freedom (nivartaka) and the path to bondage (pravartaka), as explained by Brahma.

27-29: The three debts of mankind and the means to overcome them.

29-40: Brahma explains how one should lead one's life in accordance with varṇāśramadharma. After explaining the essence of yoga, Brahma himself recedes into a state of yoga.

41-42: Gārgī's request to Yājñavalkya to further explain the enlightenment that should accompany action.

43-45: Yājñavalkya's replies that enlightenment is possible only through yoga, and yoga has eight limbs. He defines yoga as the union of the self (jīvātmā) and the Divine (paramātmā).

46-50: The eight limbs of yoga and the number of divisions in each limb.

50-70: Description of the ten yamas.

Chapter I

1-5: The qualities of sage Yājñavalkya.

yājñavalkyaṁ muniśreṣṭhaṁ sarvajñaṁ jñānanirmalam |
sarvaśāstrārthatatvajñaṁ sadā dhyānaparāyaṇam ||1||
vedavedāṅgatatvajñaṁ yogeṣu pariniṣṭhitam |
jitendriyaṁ jitakrodhaṁ jitāhāraṁ jitāmayam ||2||
tapasvinaṁ jitāmitraṁ brahmaṇyaṁ brāhmaṇapriyam |
tapovanagataṁ saumyaṁ sandhyopāsanatatparam ||3||
brahmavidbhirmahābhāgairbrāhmaṇaiśca samāvṛtam |
sarvabhūtasamaṁ śāntaṁ satyasandhaṁ gataklamam ||4||
guṇajñaṁ sarvabhūteṣu parārthaikaprayojanam |
bruvantaṁ paramātmānamṛṣīṇāmugratejasām ||5|

Yājñavalkya, the doyen among sages, all-knowing, of pure and unsullied knowledge, having realized the essence of all the Vedic scriptures (śāstra-s), abiding in meditation, having understood the essence of the Vedas and Vedangas,[1] with absolute mastery over the different aspects of yoga and

---

[1] The Vedas and the vedāṅgas. The Vedas are called "sanātana dharma." If we were to envision the Divine in a human form, the Vedas would be the "breath of the Divine." Just as the breath is inseparable from humans, the Vedas were considered inseparable from the Divine. Four Vedas are presently available: the Ṛg Veda, Yajur Veda, Sāma Veda, and Atharva Veda.

In order to understand the Vedas, one must study of the vedāṅgas. The word "aṅga" means "limb." The vedāṅgas or limbs of the Vedas are six:

1. śikṣā - Vedic phonetics

2. vyākaraṇa - grammar

3. nirukta - etymological explanations of the Vedic words

4. jyotiṣa - astronomy

5. kalpa - details of Vedic rituals

6. chandas - prosody, various meters of composition

complete control over his senses and food,[2] devoid of anger and free from all disease, always in deep penance, having overcome all his enemies,[3] residing in a hermitage in the forest, respected and revered by brahmins[4] performing all the duties prescribed in the Vedas, gentle, attentive to the

---

These limbs can be conceived in the form of a human: śikṣā forms the nose, vyākaraṇa the face or mouth, kalpa the hands, nirukta the ears, chandas the feet, and jyotiṣa the eyes.

This metaphor has significance. The first limb, śikṣā or Vedic phonetics, is the nose, not because of the associated sense of smell, but because we breathe through our nose, and the breath sustains our life. Phonetics is the life sustaining breath of the Vedic mantras.

The second limb, vyākaraṇa or Vedic grammar, is the mouth–the mouth is critical to speak any language, as is grammar.

The third limb, nirukta, is the dictionary for the Vedic language. It deals with the derivation of words, their roots and meanings–the etymology of the Vedic language. It is equated to the ears, because it is through the ears that language with all its meaning reaches us.

The fourth limb, jyotiṣa or astronomy, is compared to the eyes. Our eyes aid us in perceiving things, close or distant. The science of astronomy help us see or calculate the right time for rituals and actions.

The fifth limb, kalpa, is equated to the hands. Just as our hands are the instruments we use to perform so many essential actions, kalpa tells how to perform the Vedic rituals based on the knowledge of the five other limbs.

The sixth limb, chandas or the art of prosody, forms the feet. The Vedas are mostly written in the form of poetry. Poetry flows well with a meter. The Vedas contain various poetic meters in which mantras are recited.

[2] According to ayurveda, a major cause of disease is "āma," the toxic result of incomplete or incorrect metabolism. Mentally too, we may accumulate toxicity; that is the āma at the psychological level. "Jita" means "conquered." Therefore "jitāmaya" refers to one who has won over both mental and physical āma.

[3] The "enemies" here are internal, called "ṣaḍūrmi" or six waves. They are kāma (desire), krodha (anger), lobha (greed), moha (delusion), mada (arrogance or ego), and mātsarya (jealousy or envy). These ceaseless waves drag us deeper into the ocean of bondage.

[4] A brahmin is one who has realized the highest truth or at least makes a determined endeavor in that direction.

regular practice of sandhyāvandana,[5] surrounded by many great realized sages, with equanimity toward all beings, at peace with himself, always mindful, the embodiment of truth, teaching the essence of the highest truth to many revered sages, recognizing and appreciating the good qualities in all beings, and transmitting the highest knowledge for the welfare of others.

6-8: Gārgī's request to Yājñavalkya to teach her the essence of yoga.

tamevaṁ guṇasaṁpannaṁ nārīṇāmuttamā vadhūḥ |
maitreyī ca mahābhāgā gārgī ca brahmavidvarā ||6||
sabhāmadhyagatā ceyamṛṣīṇāmugratejasām |
praṇamya daṇḍavadbhūmau gārgyetadvākyamabravīt ||7||
gārgyuvāca--
bhagavansarvaśāstrajña sarvabhūtahite rata |
yogatatvaṁ mama brūhi sāṅgopāṅgaṁ vidhānataḥ ||8||

In the assembly of great sages, the wife of Yājñavalkya, known as Gārgī, endowed with unparalleled qualities, seeking the highest truth, prostrated[6] and spoke as follows.

Gārgī said, "Revered one, who has studied and realized the essence of the śāstras, and is concerned about the welfare of all beings, please teach me the essence of yoga with all its branches and sub-branches."[7]

---

[5] Sandhyāvandana is a ritual done thrice a day, in the morning, afternoon and evening. Meditation on the gāyatri mantra and the practice of prāṇāyāma form an intrinsic part of this ritual. Sandhyāvandana is referenced several times in this text. (See Chapter 6, for example.)

[6] The Sanskrit word for the act of prostration is "namaskāra." The two syllables, na and ma, mean "not mine" while "kāra" is derived from the root "kṛ" to do. The act of prostration indicates an attitude of surrender and letting go.

[7] The word "sa" means "with." Thus sāṅgopāṅga means to study the Vedas with all its limbs (aṅgas) and auxiliary limbs (upāṅgas). The four Vedas and six vedāṅgas have been listed. There are four upāṅgas: theory of rituals (mīmāmsā), science of logic (nyāya), spiritual parables and stories (purāṇa), and rules of ethical conduct (dharmaśāstra).

9-19: Yājñavalkya meditates on the Divine (in the form of Nārāyaṇa) and describes how he approached the Creator (Brahmā), to learn the highest truth.

evaṁ pṛṣṭaḥ sa bhagavānsabhāmadhye striyā tayā |
ṝṣīnālokya netrābhyāṁ vākyametadabhāṣata ||9||
yājñavalkya uvāca --
uttiṣṭhottiṣṭha bhadraṁ te gārgi brahmavidāṁ vare |
vakṣyāmi yogasarvasvaṁ brahmaṇā kīrtitaṁ purā ||10||
samāhitamanā gārgi śṛṇu tvaṁ gadato mama |
ityuktvā brahmavicchreṣṭho yājñavalkyastaponidhiḥ ||11||
nārāyaṇaṁ jagannāthaṁ sarvabhūtahṛdi sthitam |
vāsudevaṁ jagadyoniṁ yogidhyeyaṁ nirañjanam ||12||
ānandamamṛtaṁ nityaṁ paramātmānamīśvaram|
dhyāyanhṛdi hṛṣīkeśaṁ manasā susamāhitaḥ ||13||
netrābhyāṁ tāṁ samalokya kṛpayā vākyamabravīt |
ehyehi gārgi sarvajñe sarvaśāstraviśārade ||14||
yogaṁ vakṣyāmi vidhivaddhātroktaṁ parameṣṭhinā |
munayaḥ śrūyatāmatra gārgyā saha samāhitāḥ ||15||
padmāsane samāsīnaṁ caturānanamavyayam |
carācarāṇāṁ sraṣṭāraṁ brahmāṇaṁ parameṣṭhinam ||16||
kadācittatra gatvāhaṁ stutvā stotraiḥ praṇamya ca |
pṛṣṭavānimamevārthaṁ yanmāṁ tvaṁ paripṛcchasi ||17||
devadeva jagannātha caturmukha pitāmaha |
yenāhaṁ yāmi nirvāṇaṁ karmaṇā mokṣamavyayam ||18||
jñānaṁ ca paramaṁ guhyaṁ yathāvadbrūhi me prabho |

Requested thus, the revered Yājñavalkya viewed all the assembled sages

---

In addition to these four, there are also four upavedas or auxiliary Vedas: the science of health (āyurveda), economics and politics (arthaśāstra), weaponry (dhanurveda), music and dance (gāndharvaveda).

and spoke: "Gārgī, best among those who have realized the ultimate truth,[8] arise. May all be well with you. I will explain the essence of yoga as it was taught [to me] by the Creator (Brahmā). Listen to me with a focused mind."

Saying thus, meditating in his heart with one-pointed concentration upon Nārāyaṇa (the Divine), the refuge of the universe, residing in the heart of all beings in all worlds, the source of this universe, worthy to be meditated upon by yogis, unattached, blissful, immortal, eternal, omnipresent, and the ruler of the senses, Yājñavalkya, rich in austerity and the greatest among the realized souls, beholding Gārgī with compassion, said, "Gārgī, realized one who is proficient in all the śāstras, come forward. I will explain the principles of yoga which were taught to me by Brahmā. Listen to me with a focused mind.

"Once I approached Brahmā, who was seated on a lotus flower, with four faces, imperishable, eternal, the creator of the world with all animate and inanimate objects, known as parameṣṭhī. Expressing my devotion and prostrating before him with reverence, I asked him about the same subject about which you ask me now.

"Lord! Protector of the universe, one who has four faces, ancestor of all humanity, please teach me the means by which I can attain nirvāṇa or mokṣa (eternal peace and freedom), that supreme enlightenment which is a closely guarded secret."

19-27: The path to freedom (nivartaka) and the path to bondage (pravartaka), as explained by Brahmā.

māmālokya prasannātmā jñānakarmāṇyabhāṣata |

---

[8] There are references in various ancient texts to women who were well-read and practiced yoga. For example, in the Ramayana, there is reference to Kausalya, Rama's mother, practicing prāṇāyāma. In this text, Yājñavalkya consistently addresses Gārgī with much respect, acknowledging her wisdom and praising her as one who has realized the highest truth.

jñānasya dvividhau jñeyau panthānau vedacoditau ||20||
anuṣṭhitau tau vidvadbhiḥ pravartakanivartakau |
varṇāśramoktaṁ yat karma kāmasaṅkalpapurvakam ||21||
pravartakaṁ bhavedetatpunarāvṛttihetukam |
kartavyamiti vidhyuktaṁ karma kāmavivarjitam ||22||
yena yatkriyate samyak jñānayuktaṁ nivartakam |
nivartakaṁ hi puruṣaṁ nivartayati janmataḥ ||23||
pravartakaṁ hi sarvatra punarāvṛttihetukam |
varṇāśramoktaṁ karmaiva vidhyuktaṁ kāmavarjitam ||24||
vidhivatkurvatastasya muktirgārgi kare sthitā |
varṇāśramoktaṁ karmaiva vidhivatkāmapūrvakam ||25||
yena yatkriyate tasya garbhavāsaḥ kare sthitaḥ |
saṁsārabhīrubhistasmātvidhyuktaṁ kāmavarjitam ||26||
vidhivat karma kartavyaṁ jñānena saha sarvadā |

Thus requested by me, Brahmā, the master and the guide of the universe, beheld me graciously and explained the means to enlightenment: "Following one's duty, with desire, is pravartaka, which is the cause for rebirth. Following the actions prescribed in the Vedas properly, devoid of desire, with the goal of englightenment, is nivartaka. It is nivartaka which releases one from rebirth. It is pravartaka which is always the cause for rebirth."

Gārgī! Freedom is in the hand of (is sure to be attained by) one doing the actions according to one's dharma, devoid of desire, as said in the Vedas. Life in the womb is in the hand of one who does the actions according to one's dharma, as said in the Vedas, with desire. Thus the actions prescribed in the Vedas must be done always, without desire, with the goal of enlightenment (jñāna) by those who fear this bondage (samsāra).

27-29: The three debts of mankind and the means to overcome them.

jātāśca triṣu lokeṣu ānulomyena mānavāḥ ||27||
te devānāmṛṣīṇāṁ ca pitṝṇāmṛṇinastathā |
ṛṣibhyo brahmacaryeṇa pitṛbhyaśca sutaistathā ||28||

kuryādyajñena devebhyaḥ svāśramaṁ dharmamācaran |

Human beings, born in all the three worlds, are naturally indebted to the devas, sages, and ancestors. By learning the Vedas [one can free oneself] from the debts of the sages; by progeny, from the debts of one's ancestors; by performing appropriate rites and rituals while following the duties of one's stage in life, (āshrama) from the devas.[9]

29-40: Brahmā explains how one should lead one's life in accordance with varṇāśramadharma. After explaining the essence of yoga, Brahmā himself recedes into a state of yoga.

catvāro brāhmaṇasyoktā āśramāḥ śruticoditāḥ ||29||
kṣatriyasya trayaḥ proktā dvāvekau vaiśyaśūdrayoḥ |
adhītya vedaṁ vedārthaṁ sāṅgopāṅgaṁ vidhānataḥ ||30||
snāyādvidhyuktamārgeṇa brahmacaryavrataṁ caran |
saṁskṛtāyāṁ savarṇāyāṁ putramutpādayettataḥ ||31||
yajedagnau tu vidhivatbhāryayā saha vā vinā |
kāntāre vijane deśe phalamūlodakānvite ||32||
tapaścaranvasennityaṁ sāgnihotraḥ samāhitaḥ |
ātmanyagnīnsamāropya sannyasedvidhinā tataḥ ||33||
sanyāsāśramasaṁyukto nityaṁ karma samācaran |
yāvatkṣetrī bhavettāvat yajedātmānamātmani ||34||
kṣatriyaśca caredevamāsanyāsāśramātsadā |
vānaprasthāśramādevaṁ caredvaiśyaḥ samāhitaḥ ||35||
śūdraḥ śuśrūṣayā nityaṁ gṛhasthāśramaṁ ācaret |
śūdrasya brahmacaryaṁ ca munibhiḥ kaiścidiṣyate ||36||
ānulomyaprasūtānāṁ trayāṇāmāśramāstrayaḥ |
śūdravacchūdrajātānāṁ ācāraḥ kīrtito budhaiḥ ||37||

---

[9] All our lives, our actions are oriented toward achieving some goal—toward attainment and acquisition. However, to attain real freedom, we must direct ourselves towards giving rather than receiving. Many rituals in the Vedas incorporate the intent and act of giving, citing our indebtedness to our ancestors, sages of the past, the Divine, our parents, teachers, nature and so on.

caturṇāmāśramasthānāmahanyahani nityaśaḥ |
vidhyuktaṁ karma kartavyaṁ kāmasaṅkalpavarjitam ||38||
tasmāttvamapi yogīndra svāśramaṁ dharmamācaran |
śraddhayā vidhivatsamyak jñānakarma samācara ||39||
iti me karmasarvasvaṁ yogarūpaṁ ca tatvataḥ |
upadiśya tato brahmā yoganiṣṭho'bhavatsvayam ||40||

According to the Vedas, four stages are laid down for a brahmin, three stages for a kṣatriya, two stages for a vaiśya, and one stage for the fourth division.

Having learnt the Vedas (in the brahmacarya-āśrama), with all its branches and sub-branches, in the proper manner, one must leave the brahmacarya-āśrama, in the prescribed manner, following the vows of brahmacarya-āśrama during the transition, and must [marry and] beget children of a chaste girl of the same division [thus entering gṛhastha-āśrama]. Then he must perform the rituals with the [three] fires as prescribed in the Vedas.

With or without his wife [in vānaprastha-āśrama], he must live in a secluded place in the forest, which has sufficient fruits, roots and water, doing penance (tapas) and daily Vedic ritual (agnihotra), with a focused mind.

He must then take sanyāsa (renunciation or monkhood) in the proper manner, having [symbolically] merged the [three] fires with his self. Following sanyāsa-āśrama, doing his duty always, as long as he possesses a body (till the end of his life), he must dissolve the mind in the self.

The actions prescribed by the Vedas must be done every day, always, without the motivation of desire, by those belonging to all the four stages in life (āśramas). The kṣatriya too must always observe these stages similarly, except sanyāsa-āśrama. A vaiśya must, with concentration, observe the stages other than vānaprastha-āśrama and sanyāsa-āśrama. The fourth division must always observe gṛhastha-āśrama, and according to some sages, brahmacarya-āśrama also.

Therefore, you too, master of yogis, performing the duties of your āśrama properly, with sincerity, in the prescribed manner, do the actions that will lead you to enlightenment.

Having thus explained the essence of karma and yoga to me, Brahmā himself receeded into a state of yoga.

41-42: Gārgī's request to Yājñavalkya to further explain the enlightenment that should accompany dutiful action.

śrutvaitadyājñavalkyoktaṁ vākyaṁ gārgī mudānvitā |
punaḥ prāha muniśreṣṭhamṛṣīmadhye varānanā ||41||
gārgyuvāca --
jñānena saha yogīndra vidhyuktaṁ karma kurvataḥ |
tvayoktaṁ muktirastīti tayorjñānaṁ vada prabho ||42||

Having heard the words of Yājñavalkya with great happiness, beautiful Gārgī again spoke thus in the midst of the sages, to the greatest among sages (Yājñavalkya). Gārgī said, "O greatest of yogis! It was stated by you that there is freedom (mukti or mokṣa) for one who does the actions (karma) prescribed in the Vedas with an enlightened mind (jñāna). Master, between the two tell us about this enlightenment."

43-45: Yājñavalkya's replies that enlightenment is possible only through yoga, and yoga has eight limbs. He defines yoga as the union of the self (jīvātmā) and the Divine (paramātmā).

bhāryayā tvevamuktastu yājñavalkyastaponidhiḥ |
tāṁ samālokya kṛpayā jñānarūpamabhāṣata ||43||
yājñavalkya uvāca--
jñānaṁ yogātmakaṁ viddhi yogaścāṣṭāṅgasaṁyutaḥ |
saṁyogo yoga ityukto jīvātmaparamātmanoḥ ||44|
vakṣyāmyaṅgāni te samyagyathā pūrvaṁ mayā śrutam |
samāhitamanā gārgī ṛṣibhiḥ saha saṁśṛṇu ||45||

Yājñavalkya, thus requested by his wife, looking upon her with kindness, explained the essence of enlightenment: "Understand that enlightenment is yoga (yoga leads to enlightenment), and yoga has eight limbs. Yoga is said to be the union of the individual self (jīvātmā) and the supreme self (divine or paramātmā). I will clearly explain the limbs to you, as they were heard by me earlier. O Gārgī! Listen to me with a focused mind along with the sages."

46-50: The eight limbs of yoga and the number of divisions in each limb.

yamaśca niyamaścaiva āsanaṁ ca tathaiva ca |
prāṇāyāmastathā gārgī pratyāhāraśca dhāraṇā ||46||
dhyānaṁ samādhiretāni yogāṅgāni varānane |
yamasca niyamaścaiva daśadhā saṁprakīrtitaḥ ||47||
āsanānyuttamānyaṣṭau trayaṁ teṣūttamottamam |
prāṇayāmastridhā proktaḥ pratyahāraśca pañcadhā ||48||
dhāraṇā pañcadhā proktā dhyānaṁ ṣoḍhā prakīrtitam |
trayaṁ teṣūttamaṁ proktaṁ samādhistvekarūpakaḥ ||49||
bahudhā kecidicchanti vistareṇa pṛthak śṛṇu |

Beautiful Gārgī! These are the limbs: yama, niyama, āsana, prāṇāyāma, pratyāhāra, dhāraṇā, dhyāna, and samādhi. Yama and niyama are sub-divided into ten types [of practices]. Eight āsanas are important and among them, three are most important. Prāṇāyāma is said to be of three types and pratyāhāra of five types. Dhāraṇā is said to be of five types. Dhyāna is of six types; among them, three are said to be more important. Samādhi is one, [but] some think it to be of many divisions.

50-70: Description of the ten yamas.

ahiṁsā satyamasteyaṁ brahmacaryaṁ dayārjavam ||50||
kṣamādhṛtirmitāhāraḥ śaucaṁ tvete yamā daśa |
karmaṇā manasā vācā sarvabhūteṣu sarvadā ||51||
akleśajananaṁ proktamahiṁsātvena yogibhiḥ |
vidhyuktaṁ cedahiṁsā syātkleśajanmaiva jantuṣu ||52||
vedenokte'pi hiṁsāsyādabhicārādi karma yat |
satyaṁ bhūtahitaṁ proktaṁ na yathārthābhibhāṣaṇam ||53||

karmaṇā manasā vācā paradravyeṣu niḥspṛhā |
asteyamiti sā proktā ṛṣibhistattvadarśibhiḥ ||54||
karmaṇā manasā vācā sarvāvasthāsu sarvadā |
sarvatra maithunatyāgo brahmacaryaṁ pracakṣate ||55||
brahmacaryāśramasthānāṁ yatīnāṁ naiṣṭikasya ca |
brahmacaryaṁ tu tatproktaṁ tathaivāraṇyavāsinām ||56||
ṛtāvṛtau svadāreṣu saṅgatiryā vidhānataḥ |
brahmacaryaṁ tu tatproktaṁ gṛhasthāśramavāsinām ||57||
rājñaścaiva gṛhasthasya brahmacaryaṁ prakīrtitam |
viśāṁ vṛttavatāṁ caiva kecidicchanti paṇḍitāḥ ||58||
śuśrūṣaiva tu śūdrasya brahmacaryaṁ prakīrtitam |
śuśrūṣā vā gurornityaṁ brahmacaryamudāhṛtam ||59||
guravaḥ pañca sarveṣāṁ caturṇāṁ śruticoditāḥ |
mātā pitā tathācāryo mātulaḥ śvaśurastathā ||60||
eṣu mukhyāstrayaḥ proktā ācāryaḥ pitarau tathā |
eṣu mukhyatamastveka ācāryaḥ paramārthavit ||61||
tamevaṁ brahmāvicchreṣṭhaṁ nityakarmaparāyaṇam |
śuśrūṣayārcayennityaṁ tuṣṭo'bhūdyena vā guruḥ ||62||
dayā ca sarvabhūteṣu sarvatrānugrahaḥ smṛtaḥ |
vihiteṣu tadanyeṣu manovākkāyakarmaṇām ||63||
pravṛttau vā nivṛttau vā ekarūpatvamārjavam |
priyāpriyeṣu sarveṣu samatvaṁ yaccharīriṇām ||64||
kṣamā saiveti vidvadbhirgaditā vedavādibhiḥ |
arthahānau ca bandhūnāṁ viyogeṣvapi sampadām ||65||
tayoḥ prāptau ca sarvatra cittasya sthāpanaṁ dhṛtiḥ |
aṣṭau grāsā munerbhakṣyāḥ ṣoḍaśāraṇyavāsinām ||66||
dvātriṁśacca gṛhasthānāṁ yatheṣṭaṁ brahmacāriṇām |
eṣāmayaṁ mitāhāro hyanyeṣāmalpabhojanam ||67||
śaucaṁ tu dvividhaṁ proktaṁ bāhyamābhyantaraṁ tathā |
mṛjjalābhyāṁ smṛtaṁ bāhyaṁ manaḥśuddhistathāntaram ||68||
manaḥśuddhiśca vijñeyā dharmeṇādhyātmavidyayā |
ātmavidyā ca dharmaśca pitrācāryeṇa vānadhe ||69||
tasmātsarveṣu kāleṣu sarvairniḥśreyasārthibhiḥ |

guravaḥ śrutasampannā mānyā vāṅmanasādibhiḥ ||70||
iti śrīyogayājñavalkye prathmo'dhyāyaḥ ||

Listen to the description of each one [of the limbs]. Ahimsā, satya, asteya, brahmacarya, dayā, ārjava, kṣamā, dhṛti, mitāhāra, and śauca are the ten yamas. Refraining from harming (creating suffering for) any living being, at all times, by thought, word, or deed is said to be ahimsā by yogis. Even actions which cause harm to other beings are ahimsā if it is mandated by the Vedas. [Harmful] actions such as rituals done with the intention of harming a foe are himsā, even if [the means for the same are] provided (not mandated) in the Vedas.

Satya is not merely speaking the plain truth, [but to say] that which is beneficial to all beings. According to sages who have realised the truth, absence of desire for others' possessions is said to be asteya.

Renouncing sex, in thought, word, or deed, at all times, all places, in all states [of mind and body], is considered brahmacarya for those in the brahmacarya-āśrama, for monks, for those committed to brahmacharya throughout their lives, and for those who are in the vānaprastha-āśrama (the third stage in life when one retires to the forest). For householders, intimacy with their wives, in the prescribed period, in the proper manner, is considered brahmacarya. [These rules of] brahmacarya are prescribed for kṣatriyas who are householders, and by some scholars for vaiśyas of good conduct as well. For the fourth division, serving one's guru is said to be brahmacarya. For everyone, serving one's guru at all times is [also] said to be brahmacarya.

For all divisions, five gurus are described in the Vedas: one's mother, father, [spiritual] teacher (ācārya), [maternal] uncle, and father-in-law. Among them, three are considered important: one's [spiritual] teacher and parents. Among them, one is most important: the [spiritual] teacher who has realized the highest truth. One must always revere this teacher, the best among those who have realised the highest truth (ultimate nature of reality), who remains committed to his daily [Vedic] duties, by performing the service that pleases him.

Dayā (kindness, compassion) is to be kind to all beings everywhere.

Equality towards all things, favourable or unfavourable, is said to be kṣamā (forbearance, forgiveness) by scholars well versed in the Vedas.

When wealth is lost or gained, when one is separated from loved ones or joined with them, steadiness of mind in all [such] situations is dhṛti.

A monk may have eight mouthfuls of food [daily], those in vānaprastha-āśrama, sixteen mouthfuls, a householder, thirty two, and students as much as they wish. This is mitāhāra (controlled diet) for them, and for others [in general], it is eating less.

Śauca (purity) is said to be of two types: external and internal. External purity is [achieved] by cleansing agents like water and [a kind of fragrant] earth (like soap). Internal purity is the purity of the mind. Purity of the mind is evidenced by the dharma (ethical values) the person follows, and the internal quest for self knowledge (spiritual search).

This quest for the knowledge of the self, or an ethical life can be inculcated only by the elders or the teacher, flawless [Gārgī]! Hence people who desire to attain freedom, must at all times, through thought, word and deed, hold in respect the great sages and teachers who have realized the eternal truths declared in the Vedas.

Chapter II

OUTLINE

1-2: List of the ten niyamas.

2-3: Definition of tapas.

3-4: Definition of santoṣa.

4: Definition of āstikya.

5: Definition of dāna.

6-7: Definition of īśvarapūjana.

8-10: Description of siddhāntaśravaṇa for each division of society.

10-11: Definition of hrī.

11: Definition of mati.

12-18: Detailed description of japa.

19: Definition of vrata.

Chapter II

1-2: List of the ten niyamas.

yājñavalkya uvaca--

tapaḥ santoṣa āstikyaṁ dānamīśvarapūjanam |

siddhāntaśravaṇaṁcaiva hrīrmatiśca japo vratam ||1||

ete tu niyamāḥ proktāstānśca sarvānpṛthak śṛṇu |

Tapas, santoṣa, āstikya, dāna, īśvarapūjana, siddhāntaśravaṇa, hrī, mati, japa, and vrata—these are the niyamas. Listen to their description one by one.

2-3: Definition of tapas.

vidhinoktena mārgeṇa kṛcchracāndrāyanādibhiḥ ||2||

śarīraśoṣaṇaṁ prāhustāpasāstapa uttamam |

Those who are well versed in tapas say that drying the body by following kṛcchra, cāndrāyana[10] etc., in accordance with the Vedas, is the best tapas.

---

[10] Kṛcchra and cāndrāyana are regimens of fasting. The word for fasting in Sanskrit is "upavāsa." "Upa" means "near" and "vas" means "to reside." Residing or staying close to the Divine or to one's self is upavāsa. Limiting food intake can facilitate this goal. A light stomach aids both prāṇāyāma and meditation; it is instrumental in focusing the mind. Fasting may help restore physical health and detoxify the body.

However, when devoid of the goal of calming and focusing the mind, such fasting is not tapas. During the period of fasting, pranayama and meditation on a mantra are helpful in reducing mental impurities (kleśas as in Yogasūtra II.3).

There are different traditional regimens of fasting. For example, one suggestion is that every eleventh day of the cycle of the moon be a day of fasting.

Cāndrāyana is another example, suggested here. This is a longer regimen, based on the waxing and waning of the moon. One starts on a full moon day; that day, fifteen measures of food are allowed. On the next day, one should take fourteen measures of food. Continuing thus, every day the adherent takes one measure of food less than the preceding day, until the new moon day, when is a day of complete fasting with only water.

3-4: Definition of santoṣa.

yadṛcchālābhato nityamalaṁ puṁso bhavediti ||3||
yā dhīstāmṛṣayaḥ prāhuḥ santoṣaṁ sukhalakṣaṇam |

"Whatever life brings is ample." This attitude [of contentment], say the sages, is santoṣa, the very definition of happiness.

4: Definition of āstikya.

dharmādharmeṣu viśvāso yastadāstikyamucyate ||4||

Trust in dharma and adharma (ethical and unethical conduct) is āstikya.

5: Definition of dāna.

nyāyārjitaṁ dhanaṁ cānnamanyadvā yatpradīyate |
arthibhyaḥ śraddhayā yuktaṁ dānametadudāhṛtam ||5||

Giving wealth, food, or other possessions that one has rightfully earned, to those in need, with sincerity is said to be dāna.[11]

6-7: Definition of īśvarapūjana.

yatprasannasvabhāvena viṣṇuṁ vā'pyanyameva vā |

Then, starting on the first day after the new moon, this regimen is reversed. Every day, the adherent takes one measure of food more than the preceding day, reaching fifteen measures of food on the full moon day. This ends the cycle.

Cāndrāyana may also be started on the day after the new moon, taking one measure of food, then increasing to fifteen, adding one measure a day, and reducing from fifteen to one measure again, reducing one measure of food every day.

It is important to note that these procedures vary for each individual based on considerations such as age and health.

[11] In dāna, as in any of the other niyamas, attitude is crucial. The Bhagavad Gita (XVII.20-22) classifies dāna into three types based on the gunas. Sātvika dāna is to give a deserving person the right thing, at the right time, at the right place, with the attitude that "this is not mine." Giving something in order to gain a favor, with show and pomp, is called rājasa dāna. Giving something at the wrong time to an unworthy person with the wrong attitude, in an insulting manner, is tāmasa dāna.

yathāśaktyarcanaṁ bhaktyā hyetadīśvarapūjanam ||6||
rāgādyapetaṁ hṛdayaṁ vāgaduṣṭānṛtavādinā |
hiṁsādirahitaḥ kāya etadīśvarapūjanam ||7||

Worshipping Viṣṇu or other deities to the extent of one's capability, with a pure and devoted mind, is īśvarapūjana. A mind devoid of desire, speech unsullied by lies and a body that does no harm [to others] is [also] īśvarapūjana.

8-10: Description of siddhāntaśravaṇa for each division of society.

siddhāntaśravaṇaṁ proktaṁ vedāntaśravaṇaṁ budhaiḥ |
dvijavatkṣatriyasyoktaṁ siddhāntaśravaṇaṁ budhaiḥ ||8||
viśāṁ ca kecidicchanti śīlavṛttavatāṁ satām |
śūdrāṇāṁ ca striyāścaiva svadharmasthatapasvinām ||9||
siddhāntaśravaṇaṁ proktaṁ purāṇaśravaṇaṁ budhaiḥ |

Listening to vedānta (the philosophy explained in the Upaniṣads, the last part of the Vedas) is said to be siddhāntaśravaṇa by the wise. For the kṣatriya, siddhāntaśravaṇa is said to be the same as for brahmins, and some say the same for vaiśyas who are possessed of good character and conduct. For the fourth division and women, who perform their duties and control their senses, listening to the purāṇas (other sacred texts which explain philosophy mixed with stories and parables) is said to be siddhāntaśravaṇa by the wise.[12]

10-11: Definition of hrī.

vedalaukikamārgeṣu kutsitaṁ karma yadbhavet ||10||
tasminbhavati yā lajjā hrīstu saiveti kīrtitā |

---

[12] The essential teaching of the Vedas were also given in the form of other texts called the itihāsas and the purāṇas. The itihāsas, such as the Rāmāyaṇa and Mahābhārata, represent the essence of the Vedas. The Rāmāyaṇa is said to be an expansion of the message of the Vedas. The Mahābhārata is called the fifth Veda. The Bhāgavata, a purāṇa, is said to be the fruit of the Vedas.

The shame that one feels at doing actions that are considered despicable by the Vedas and by the ways of the world is called hrī.[13]

11: Definition of mati.

vihiteṣu ca sarveṣu śraddhā yā sā matirbhavet ||11||

Sincerity in all the duties laid down [in the Vedas] is mati.

12-18: Detailed description of japa.

guruṇā copadiṣṭo'pi vedabāhyavivarjitaḥ |
vidhinoktena mārgeṇa mantrābhyāso japaḥ smṛtaḥ ||12||
adhītya vedaṁ sūtraṁ vā purāṇaṁ setihāsakam |
eteṣvabhyasanaṁ yacca tadabhyāso japaḥ smṛtaḥ ||13||
japaśca dvividhaḥ prokto vāciko mānasastathā |
vācika upāṁśuruccaiśca dvividhaḥ parikīrtitataḥ ||14||
mānaso mananadhyānabhedād dvaividhyamāsthitaḥ |
uccairjapādupāṁśuśca sahasraguṇa ucyate ||15||
mānasastu tathopāṁśoḥ sahasraguṇa ucyate |
mānasācca tathā dhyānaṁ sahastraguṇamucyate ||16||
uccairjapastu sarveṣāṁ yathoktaphalado bhavet |
nīcaiḥ śruto na cetso'pi śrutaścenniṣphalo bhavet ||17||
ṛṣiṁ chando'dhidaivaṁ ca dhyāyanmantraṁ ca sarvadā |
yastu mantrajapo gārgi sa eva hi phalapradaḥ ||18||

Repeating, in the proper manner, the Vedic mantra, into which one has been initiated by the guru is considered japa. Constantly reading and reflecting upon the Vedas, purāṇas, itihāsas or sūtras after studying them—such a practice is also called japa.

Japa is of two types: verbal and mental. Verbal japa is said to be of two types: aloud and soft. Mental japa is classified into two types: silent repetition (manana) and uninterrupted meditation (dhyāna).

---

[13] Hrī implies clarity of conscience to distinguish between what shall, and what shall not, be done.

Soft verbal japa is said to be thousand times more beneficial than the verbal japa done aloud. Silent repetition (manana) is said to be thousand times more beneficial than the soft verbal japa. Uninterrupted meditation (dhyāna) is said to be thousand times more beneficial than silent repetition (manana).

Loud recitation bestows the appropriate (desired) results on everybody, if not heard by those of low mentality, but if heard [by them], it becomes fruitless. The japa on a mantra in which one pays attention to the meter (chandas), the seer of the mantra (ṛṣi), and the deity depicted by it (devatā), and the mantra [itself]—such a mantrajapa alone, O Gārgī, will yield the [desired] benefits.

19: Definition of vrata.

prasannaguruṇā pūrvamupadiṣṭaṁ tvanujñayā |
dharmārthamātmasiddhyarthamupāyagrahaṇaṁ vratam ||19||
iti śrīyogayajñavalkye dvitīyo'dhyāyaḥ |

Following [with steadiness] the path of ethical conduct, toward prosperity and spiritual freedom, with the prior approval and initiation from the guru, is vrata.

Chapter III

OUTLINE

1-2: List of the eight āsanas to be discussed in this chapter.

3: Svastikāsana.

4-5: Variation of svastikāsana.

5-6: Gomukhāsana.

6-7: Padmāsana.

8: Vīrāsana.

9-11: Simhāsana.

13: Muktāsana.

14: Variation of muktāsana.

15-16: Mayūrāsana.

17-18: Instruction to Gārgī.

Chapter III

1-2: List of the eight āsanas to be discussed in this chapter.

yājñavalkya uvāca--
āsanānyadhunā vakṣye śṛṇu gārgi tapodhane |
svastikaṁ gomukhaṁ padmaṁ vīraṁ siṁhāsanaṁ tathā ||1||
bhadraṁ muktāsanaṁ caiva mayūrāsanameva ca |
tathaiteṣāṁ varārohe pṛthagvakṣyāmi lakṣaṇam ||2||

Yājñavalkya said:
Now, I will describe the āsanas. Gārgī, rich in austerity, listen to me. Svastikāsana, gomukhāsana, padmāsana, vīrāsana, simhāsana, bhadrāsana, muktāsana and mayūrāsana. I will describe these [āsanas] one by one.

3: Svastikāsana.

jānorvorantare samyakkṛtvā pādatale ubhe |
ṛjukāyaḥ sukhāsīnaḥ svastikaṁ tatpracakṣate ||3||

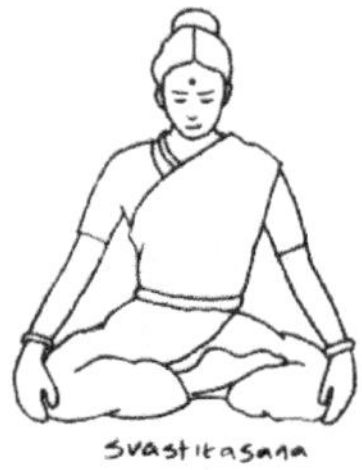

Svastikasana

Having correctly placed the soles of both the feet between the thighs and knees, one should sit (comfortably) balanced and straight-bodied. This is called svastikāsana.[14]

4-5: Variation of svastikāsana.

sīvanyāstvātmanaḥ pārśve gulphau nikṣipya pādayoḥ |
savye dakṣiṇagulphaṁ tu dakṣiṇe dakṣiṇetaram ||4||
etacca svastikaṁ proktaṁ sarvapāpapraṇāśanam |

The ankles must be placed on either side of the perineum, the left ankle on the right side and the right ankle on the left side. This too is known as

[14] The same descriptions are used by later yoga texts. See, for example: Haṭhayogapradīpikā (I.19), Gheraṇḍa Samhitā (II.13), and the Śiva Samhitā (III.95).

svastikāsana and it destroys all impurities.

5-6: Gomukhāsana.

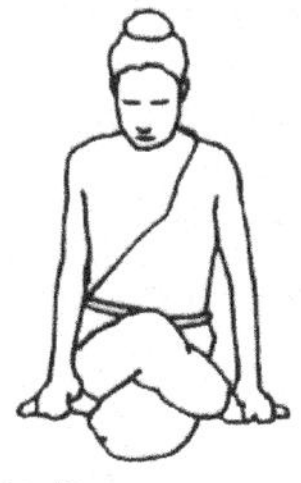

Gomukhasana

savye dakṣiṇagulphaṁ tu pṛṣṭhapārśve niyojayet ||5||
dakṣiṇe'pi tathā savyaṁ gomukhaṁ gomukhaṁ yathā |

Place the right ankle beside the buttock, on the left, and the left [ankle] at the right. This is gomukhāsana, resembling the face of a cow.[15]

6-7: Padmāsana.

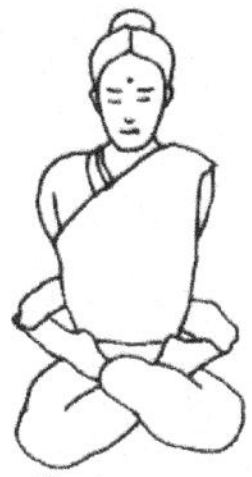

Padmasana

aṅguṣṭhau ca nibadhnīyāddhastābhyāṁ vyutkrameṇa ca ||6||
urvorupari viprendre kṛtvā pādatale ubhe |
padmāsanaṁ bhavedetatsarveṣāmapi pūjitam ||7||

The big toes must be held from behind and the feet should be placed on the (opposite) thighs. This is padmāsana which is revered by all.

8: Vīrāsana.

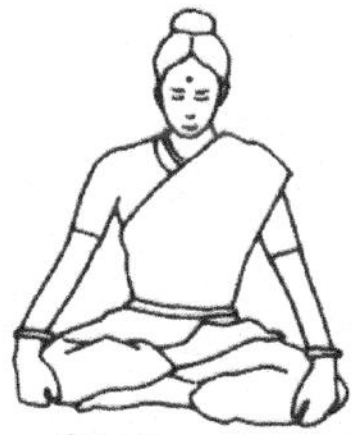

Virasana

ekaṁ pādamathaikasminvinyasyoruṇi saṁsthitam |
itarasmiṁstathā coruṁ vīrāsanamudāhṛtam ||8||

Place one foot firmly on the one thigh and the [other] thigh on the other foot. This is called vīrāsana.[16]

9-11: Simhāsana.

gulphau ca vṛṣaṇasyādhaḥ sīvanyāḥ pārśvayoḥ kṣipet |
dakṣiṇaṁ savyagulphena dakṣiṇena tathetaram ||9||
hastau ca jānvoḥ saṁsthāpya svāṅgulīśca prasārya ca |

---

[15] For similar descriptions, refer Haṭhayogapradīpikā (I.20) and Gheraṇḍa Samhitā (II.16).

[16] Refer Haṭhayogapradīpikā (I.21) for a similar description.

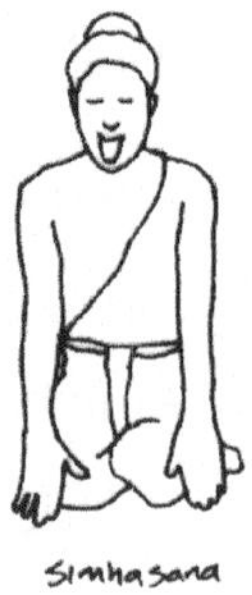
Simhasana

vyāttavaktro nirīkṣeta nāsāgraṁ susamāhitaḥ ||10||
siṁhāsanaṁ bhavedetatpūjitaṁ yogibhiḥ sadā |

Place the ankles below the scrotum, on the sides of the perineum, the left ankle on the right and the right ankle on the other side (left). Place the palms upon the knees and spread out the fingers. With an opened mouth, look at the tip of the nose with a concentrated mind. This is simhāsana,[17] always held in high esteem by yogis.

11-12: Bhadrāsana.

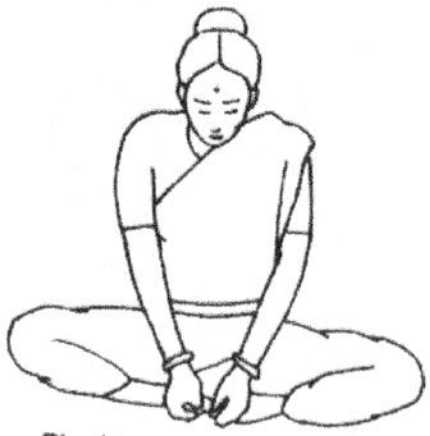
Bhadrasana

gulphau ca vṛṣṇasyādhaḥ sīvanyāḥ pārśvayoḥ kṣipet ||11||
pārśvapādau ca pāṇibhyāṁ dṛḍhaṁ buddhavā suniścalam |
bhadrāsanaṁ bhavedetatsarvavyādhiviṣāpaham ||12||

Hold firmly with the hands the feet which are on their sides and remain motionless. This is bhadrāsana, which destroys all diseases and toxins.

13: Muktāsana.

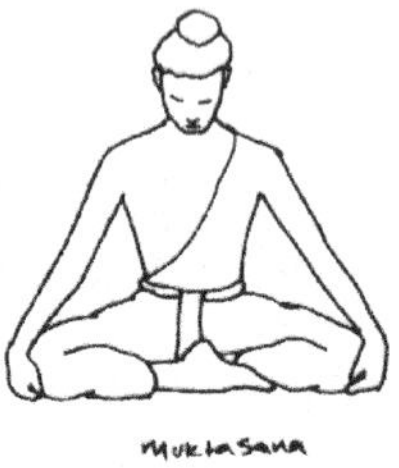
Muktasana

saṁpīḍaya sīvanīṁ sūkṣmāṁ gulphenaiva tu savyataḥ |
savyaṁ dakṣiṇagulphena muktāsanamitīritam ||13||

Press the perineum by the left ankle, and the left ankle by the right ankle—this is known as muktāsana.

14: Variation of muktāsana.

meḍhrādupari nikṣipya savyaṁ gulphaṁ tathopari |
gulphāntaraṁ ca nikṣipya muktāsanamidaṁ tu vā ||14||

Placing the left ankle above the generative organ and placing the other ankle above it is muktāsana.

[17] Refer Haṭhayogapradīpikā (I.50-52) for similar descriptions.

15-16: Mayūrāsana.

avaṣṭabhya dharāṁ samyak talābhyāṁ tu karadvayoḥ |
hastayoḥ kūrparau cāpi sthāpayannābhipārśvayoḥ ||15||
samunnataśiraḥpādo daṇḍavadvyomni saṁsthitaḥ |
mayūrāsanametattu sarvapāpapraṇāśanam ||16||

Placing the palms of the hands firmly on the ground and keeping the elbows at the side of the navel with the head and legs raised, staying in space [off the ground]—this is mayūrāsana which destroys all impurities.

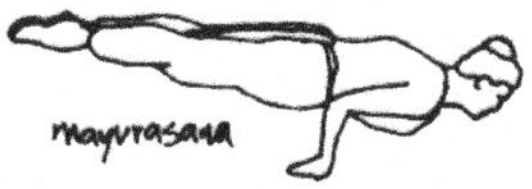

17-18: Instruction to Gārgī.

sarve cābhyantarā rogā vinaśyanti viṣāṇi ca |
yamaiśca niyamaiścaiva āsanaiśca susaṁyutā ||17||
nāḍīśuddhiṁ ca kṛtvā tu prāṇāyāmaṁ tataḥ kuru ||18||
iti śrīyogayājñavalkye tṛtīyo'dhyāyaḥ |

All internal diseases and toxins are destroyed [by the practice of āsana]. Combining yama, niyama, and āsanas, after purifying the nāḍis, do prāṇāyāma.

Appendix to Chapter III

Classical Sanskrit yoga texts quote different numbers of āsanas. For example, the Dhyānabindu Upaniṣad says, "There are as many āsanas as there are varieties of living beings." The Haṭhayogapradīpikā (I.33) says there are 84 āsanas. Gheraṇḍa Samhitā (II.1) says there are 8.4 million āsanas but, of these, 84 are the best and, of these, 32 are described (II.2) in the text. The Śiva Samhitā (III.84) says there are 84 āsanas, and out of those, four are described in the text. The same āsanas may be described by these texts under different names.

All these later yoga texts mentioned above have borrowed the descriptions of these āsanas from this text of Yājñavalkya. In fact, Yājñavalkya is quoted in many of these texts as one of the ancient sages.

For example, under the Haṭhayogapradīpikā (I.18), Brahmānanda, the commentator, mentions that the āsanas described there are approved by the sage Yājñavalkya.

Similarly, the Haṭhayogapradīpikā (II.37) says, "Some teachers say that all impurities (of the nāḍīs) are removed by prāṇāyāma alone and other acts (kriyās or cleansing techniques) are not accepted by great sages." The commentator Brahmānanda again notes that the "great sages" here includes those such as Yājñavalkya. The reader may observe that the Yoga Yājñavalkya does not describe the kriyās.

In this chapter, Yājñavalkya describes eight āsanas and variations of two of them. Of these, three are considered particularly important. The chapter ends with a note that proper practice of āsanas, along with yama and niyama, destroys diseases.

Students of yoga should note that all these texts describe only a final, classical āsana, but none of the intermediate or preparatory āsanas. Krishnamacharya would emphasize that the practice of āsanas was to be learned under the personal guidance and supervision of a teacher. The teacher has a responsibility to guide the student, selecting and modifying the āsanas according to each student's health, age, fitness, and psychology. (The reader may refer to other books by the same author—*Yoga for Body, Breath, and Mind*; *Yoga Therapy*; and *Krishnamacharya* for more details.)

Yājñavalkya mentions the removal of internal diseases as one benefit of āsanas. This does not refer only to bodily ailments. It also implies a focused and quiet mind.

The Haṭhayogapradīpikā (I.17) says that "āsana leads to steadiness, lightness of the body, and freedom from disease." The commentary then explains "steadiness" as calmness of mind arising from reducing the disturbance of rajas or uncontrolled activity, and "lightness of the body" as arising from reduction of the clouding of tamas or the inertia and heaviness in the body and mind.

Thus, "freedom from disease," as explained in the commentary is not merely a physical goal, but also related to reduction in the disturbances in the mind. The Yogasūtra (II.48) also states that the practice of āsana leads to a state of being unaffected by opposites (pleasure or pain, happiness or sorrow), which is a psychological goal too.

Thus it is clear that āsanas were not only a path to physical health in the ancient times, but also aimed at leading to calmness of the mind.

Chapter IV

OUTLINE

1-6: Gārgī's request to learn about nādīs and their positions, vāyus and their functions, and purification of the nāḍīs (nāḍīśuddhi).

6-8: Concept of prāṇa and its dispersion.

9-10: The importance of centering the prāṇa.

11-15: Description and location of the seat of the internal fire in the body (dehamadhya).

16-17: Position, shape, and size of the kandasthāna.

18-20: Position and description of the abode of the prāṇa and the jīva (nābhicakra).

21-23: Position and nature of the kuṇḍalinī.

23-24: Kuṇḍalinī and prāṇa—awakening of the kuṇḍalinī.

25-28: The 14 important nāḍīs, and the most important ones among them.

29-31: The location and features of suṣumnā nāḍī.

31-34: The relative position and features of iḍā and piṅgalā nāḍīs.

35-38: The relative position of the remaining nāḍīs.

39-46: The origin and termination of the nāḍīs.

47-49: The ten vāyus—prāṇa to dhananjaya.

50-51: The abode of prāṇa.

52-53: The abode of apāna.

54: The abode of vyāna.

55: The abode of udāna.

55-57: The abode of samāna.

58: The abode of the other five vāyus.

58-66: The process of digestion and assimilation of food and the role of the vāyus in this process.

67-71: The function of each vāyu.

71-72: Instruction to Gārgī to perform nāḍīśodhana.

Chapter IV

1-6: Gārgī's request to learn about nādīs and their positions, vāyus and their functions, and purification of the nāḍīs (nāḍīśuddhi).

śrutvaitadbhāṣitaṁ vākyaṁ yājñavalkyasya dhīmataḥ |
punaḥ prāha mahābhāgā sabhāmadhye tapasvanī ||1||
gārgyuvāca--
bhagavanbrūhi me svāminnāḍīśuddhiṁ vidhānataḥ |
kenopāyena śuddhāḥ syurnāḍayaḥ sarvadehinām ||2||
utpattiṁ cāpi nāḍīnāṁ cāraṇaṁ ca yathāvidhi |
kandaṁ ca kīdṛśaṁ proktaṁ kati tiṣṭhanti vāyavaḥ ||3||
sthānāni caiva vāyūnāṁ karmāṇi ca pṛthakpṛthak |
vijñātavyāni yānyasmindehe dehabhṛtāṁ vara ||4||
vaktumarhasi tatsarvaṁ tvatto vettā na vidyate |
ityukto bhāryayā tatra samyak tadgatamānasaḥ ||5||
gārgīṁ tāṁ susamālokya tatsarvaṁ samabhāṣata |

Having listened to the words of the wise Yājñavalkya in the assembly of sages, blessed and austere Gārgī spoke again.

Gārgī said, "Revered master, tell me in an orderly manner about the purification of the nāḍīs.[18] In the proper manner, [please explain] how the nāḍīs of all beings may be purified, the origin of the nāḍīs and their distribution, the nature of kandasthāna, the number of vāyus [in the body], the location of the vāyus and their functions, one by one—whatever may be known in this body, you, highest among beings, are most qualified to tell us about all of them. There is no one as knowledgeable as you."

Thus addressed by his wife, his mind absorbed in her question, looking at Gārgī, he (Yājñavalkya) explained all that [she asked].

---

[18] We have retained the Sanskrit term, nāḍī, for accuracy. Nāḍīs are subtle channels or meridians along which prāṇa, the life-force or energy, flows.

6-8: Concept of prāṇa and its dispersion.

yājñavalkya uvāca--
śarīraṁ tāvadevaṁ hi ṣaṇṇavatyaṅgulātmakam ||6||
viddhyetatsarvajantūnāṁ svāṅjulībhiriti priye |
śarīrādadhikaḥ prāṇo dvādaśāṅgulamānataḥ ||7||
caturdaśāṅgulaṁ kecidvadanti munisattamāḥ |
dvādaśāṅgula eveti vadanti jñānino narāḥ ||8||

Yājñavalkya said:

Beloved! Know that the body of all beings is exactly ninety six aṅgulas[19] by their own fingers. The prāṇa exceeds the body by twelve aṅgulas. Some venerable sages say [that it is] fourteen aṅgulas. [But] the realized ones say [that it is] only twelve aṅgulas.

9-10: The importance of centering the prāṇa.

ātmasthamanilaṁ vidvānātmasthenaiva vahninā |
yogābhyāsena yaḥ kuryātsamaṁ vā nyūnameva vā ||9||
sa eva brahmavicchreṣṭhaḥ sa sampūjyo narottamaḥ |
ātmasthavahninaiva tvaṁ yogajena dvijottame ||10||

The learned person who, by the practice of yoga, with the help of the fire

---

[19] An "aṅgula" is a measurement of length based on the width of the fingers. The width of four fingers, excluding the thumb, is four aṅgulas. Naturally, the span of four fingers which measures four aṅgulas is different for each individual. You will find that your height is around twenty-four times the span of four finger widths, that is, ninety-six aṅgulas.

The distances between the different important centers in the body is stated in aṅgulas, as the reader will note later in this chapter. The distances between the vital points of the body (marmasthānas) in the Chapter VII are also detailed in aṅgulas. Later yoga texts measure the distances between the cakras as well in aṅgulas.

It is interesting to note the similarity to ancient Chinese measurements: four angulas is equivalent to three cuns. The measurement of the body, seventy-two cuns, corresponds to three-fourths of ninety-six aṅgulas.

(agni)[20] equalizes or reduces the prāṇa that is within oneself, is the greatest among those who have realized the highest. He is the best among men and is fit to be worshipped. You too [Gārgī], with the help of the fire born out of yoga, master the prāṇa within oneself, by the practice of yoga.

11-15: Description and location of the seat of the internal fire in the body (dehamadhya).

ātmasthaṁ mātariśvānaṁ yogābhyāsena nirjaya |
dehamadhye śikhisthānaṁ taptajāmbūnadaprabham ||11||
trikoṇaṁ manujānāṁ ca caturasraṁ catuṣpadām |
maṇḍalaṁ tatpataṅgānāṁ satyametadbravīmi te ||12||
tanmadhye tu śikhā tanvī sadā tiṣṭhati pāvakī |
dehamadhyaṁ ca kutreti śrotumicchasi cecchṛṇu ||13||
gudāttu dvayaṅgulādūrdhvamadho meḍhrācca dvyaṅgulāt |
dehamadhyaṁ tayormadhyaṁ manuṣyāṇāmitīritam ||14||
catuṣpadāṁ tu hṛnmadhyaṁ tiraścāṁ tundamadhyamam |
dvijānāṁ tu varārohe tundamadhyamitīritam ||15||

In the center of the body is the abode of the fire, glowing like melted gold, [in the shape of] a triangle in humans, a square in animals and a circle in birds. This is the truth which I say to you. In the midst of this there is always present a fine flame. If you wish to know where the center of the body (dehamadhya) is, listen.

In humans, it is said to be two aṅgulas above the anus and two aṅgulas below the generative organ, situated in between them. In quadrupeds, it is

---

[20] The word agni (translated here as "fire") may be derived as "that which reduces everything to its end or final form." That is, agni is that which burns and reduces everything to ash finally. In Vedic thought, agni symbolizes the Divine. Just as agni burns impurities, the Divine can burn the impurities within us—the kleśas or impurities of ignorance and ego—thus leading us to our ultimate, true form as consciousness. Hence, the agni referred to here is not physical fire. Thus, later in this text, you will find reference to meditation on the Divine in the form of agni (see IX.18-24).

the center of the heart, and for other animals it is the center of the belly. For birds, it is said to be the middle of the belly, beautiful [Gārgī]!

16-17: Position, shape, and size of the kandasthāna.

kandasthānāṁ manuṣyāṇāṁ dehamadhyānnavāṅgulam |
caturaṅgulamutsedhamāyāmaśca tathāvidhaḥ ||16||
aṇḍākṛtivadākāraṁ bhūṣitaṁ tattvagādibhiḥ |
catuṣpadāṁ tiraścāṁ ca dvijānāṁ tundamadhyame ||17||

The kandasthāna of humans is nine aṅgulas from the dehamadhya. It is four aṅgulas in height and the same in width, its form is similar to the shape of an egg and is ornamented (surrounded) by the five elements of creation and sustenance (tattvas). In quadrupeds, birds and other beings, it (the kandasthāna) is in the center of the belly.

18-20: Position and description of the abode of the prāṇa and the jīva (nābhicakra).

tanmadhyaṁ nābhirityuktaṁ nābhau cakrasamudbhavaḥ |
dvādaśārayutaṁ tacca tena dehaḥ pratiṣṭhitaḥ ||18||
cakre'sminbhramate jīvaḥ pāpapuṇyapracoditaḥ |
tantupañjaramadhyasthā yathā bhramati lūtikā ||19||
jīvasya mūlacakre'sminnadhaḥ prāṇaścaratyasau |
prāṇārūḍho bhavejjīvaḥ sarvebhūteṣu sarvadā ||20||

The middle of this (the kandasthāna) is called the nābhi (navel). In the nābhi arises a cakra. That [cakra] has twelve spokes and it is by this that the body is held.[21] Just as a spider moves around in its [self-spun] cage of

---

[21] The cakra at the navel is the center for the origin of all the nāḍīs. Therefore, Patanjali (Yogasūtra III.29) says "nābhicakre kāyavyūha jñānam," that is, by samyama on the nābhi cakra, one can understand the vyūha or the arrangement of the structures of the body.

thread (web),[22] the self (jīva), instigated by his good and bad deeds, moves around in this cakra. In the lower part of this cakra, which is the base for the self (jīva), this prāṇa moves. The jīva is mounted on the prāṇa at all times in all beings.

21-23: Position and nature of the kuṇḍalinī.

tasyordhvaṁ kuṇḍalīsthānaṁ nābhestiryagathordhvataḥ |
aṣṭaprakṛtirūpā sā aṣṭadhā kuṇḍalīkṛtā ||21||
yathāvadvāyusañcāraṁ jalānnādīni nityaśaḥ |
paritaḥ kandapārśveṣu niruddhyaiva sadā sthitā ||22||
mukhenaiva samāveṣṭya brahmarandhramukhaṁ tathā |

Above this is the location of the kuṇḍalinī, all around the nābhi. Her[23] nature is of the eight aspects of the Seen[24] and her form is spiral. Obstructing the proper movement of the prāṇa, water, food, etc. from all directions, from all sides of the kandasthāna at all times, the kuṇḍalinī is present covering the opening of the the door to freedom (brahmarandhra) with her mouth.[25]

---

[22] The web of the spider is self-spun, as is the web of our own past actions. Our past actions have conditioned us, and this conditioning is responsible for our bondage.

[23] The Sanskrit word "kuṇḍalinī" is feminine in gender. Kuṇḍalinī represents the Mother Goddess and her power. She is called Śakti, or power, for she holds power over Seen (prakṛti, or the mind and world around us). The literal meaning of the word kuṇḍalinī is "spiral" or "winding in shape."

[24] The eight aspects of Seen (prakṛti) are the five forms of matter (earth, water, fire, air and space), the mind, the intellect, and the ego. The same eight aspects of prakṛti are listed in the Bhagavad Gita (VII.4).

[25] The kuṇḍalinī blocking or covering the opening to the brahmarandhra (the door to freedom) at the bottom of the suṣumnā nāḍī, refers to the Seen (prakṛti), binding the Seer and blocking its way to freedom. Bound to the Seen, the Seer is unable to ascend to its true abode at the brahmarandra.

23-24: Kuṇḍalinī and prāṇa—awakening of the kuṇḍalinī.

yogakāle tvapānena prabodhaṁ yāti sāgninā ||23||
sphurantī hṛdayākāśe nāgarūpā mahojjvalā |
vāyurvāyusakhenaiva tato yāti suṣumṇayā ||24||

It (the kuṇḍalinī) is awakened during the practice of yoga by the apāna [vāyu] along with the fire, throbbing, shining brightly in the form of a snake in the internal space (hṛdayākāśa). Then the prāṇa with (by the help of)[26] agni goes [up] by the suṣumnā.

25-28: The 14 important nāḍīs, and the most important ones among them.

kandamadhye sthitā nāḍī suṣumṇeti prakīrtitā |
tiṣṭhanti paritaḥ sarvāścakre'sminnāḍīsaṁjñakāḥ ||25||
nāḍīnāmapi sarvāsāṁ mukhyāstvetāścaturdaśa |
iḍā ca piṅgalā caiva suṣumṇā ca sarasvatī ||26||
vāruṇī caiva pūṣā ca hastijihvā yaśasvinī |
viśvodarā kuhūścaiva śaṅkhinī ca payasvinī ||27||
alambuṣā ca gāndhārī mukhyāścaitāścaturdaśa |
āsāṁ mukhyatamāstistrastisṛṣvekottamottamā ||28||

The nāḍī situated in the middle of the kandasthāna is called suṣumnā. In this [nābhi] cakra, on all the sides, are present the nāḍīs.

Among all the nāḍīs, the important ones are these fourteen: iḍā, piṅgalā, suṣumnā, sarasvatī, vāruṇī, pūṣā, hastijihvā, yaśasvinī, visvodara, kuhū, śaṅkhinī, payasvinī, alambuṣā and gāndhārī.

The brahmarandhra is the abode of the Seer, and of the Divine. The abode of the Seer and the Divine are considered the same since realizing the true nature of one's self is the same as union with the Divine. Therefore, Yājñavalkya states that yoga is the union of the Self and the Divine.

[26] Refer to VI.69-71, where Yājñavalkya mentions the role of the agni in arousing the kuṇḍalinī.

Among these, three are most important and among the three, one is the greatest.

29-31: The location and features of suṣumnā nāḍī.

kandasya madhyame gārgi suṣumṇā supratiṣṭhitā ||29||
pṛṣṭhamadhye sthitā nāḍī sā hi mūrdhni vyavasthitā |
muktimārgaḥ suṣumṇā sā brahmarandhreti kīrtitā ||30||
avyaktā saiva vijñeyā sūkṣmā sā vaiṣṇavī smṛtā |
muktimārgeti sā proktā suṣumṇā viśvadhāriṇī |

Gārgī, the suṣumnā is firmly established in the middle of the kandasthāna. That nāḍī is situated in the [center of the] back (spine) and ends in the top of the head.

That suṣumnā is the path to freedom and is called brahmarandhra (door to the Brahman). Called vaiṣṇavī, [this suṣumnā] should be known as being unmanifest and subtle. It is said to be the door to freedom (mokṣa) and the support of the universe.

31-34: The relative position and features of iḍā and piṅgalā nāḍīs.

iḍā ca piṅgalā caiva tasyāḥ savye ca dakṣiṇe ||31||
iḍā tasyāḥ sthitā savye dakṣiṇe piṅgalā sthitā |
iḍāyāṁ piṅgalāyāṁ ca carataścandrabhāskarau ||32||
iḍāyāṁ candramā jñeyaḥ piṅgalāyāṁ raviḥ smṛtaḥ |
candrastāmasa ityuktaḥ sūryo rājasa ucyate ||33||
viṣabhāgo raverbhāgaḥ somabhāgo'mṛtaṁ smṛtam |
tāveva dhattaḥ sakalaṁ kālaṁ rātridivātmakam ||34||

Iḍā and piṅgalā are on its left and right. The iḍā is situated on its left and the piṅgalā on the right. The moon and sun move in the iḍā and piṅgalā. The moon should be known [as being] in iḍā. The sun is said to be in piṅgalā. The moon is said to be tāmasic and the sun is said to be rājasic. The poisonous part is the part of the sun. The part of the moon is said to be nectar (amṛta). These two support all of time in the form of night and day.

35-38: The relative position of the remaining nāḍīs.

bhoktrī suṣumṇā kālasya guhyametadudāhṛtam |
sarasvatī kuhuścaiva suṣumṇāpārśvayoḥ sthite ||35||
gāndhārī hastijihvā ca iḍāyāḥ pṛṣṭhapārśvayoḥ |
kuhośca hastijihvāyā madhye viśvodarā sthitā ||36||
yaśasvinyāḥ kuhormadhye vāruṇī ca pratiṣṭhitā |
pūṣāyāśca sarasvatyāḥ sthitā madhye payasvinī ||37||
gāndhāryāśca sarasvatyāḥ sthitā madhye ca śaṅkhinī |
alambuṣā ca viprendre kandamadhyādadhaḥ sthitā ||38||

Suṣumnā engulfs time.[27] This is said to be a secret.

Sarasvatī and kuhu are situated along the sides of the suṣumnā.

Gāndhārī and hastijihva are at the back and side of iḍā.

Visvodarā is situated between kuhu and hastijihvā.

Vāruṇī is situated between yaśasvinī and kuhu.

Payasvinī is situated between pūṣā and sarasvatī.

In between gāndhārī and sarasvatī is situated śaṅkhinī.

Alambuṣā is situated below the center of the kandasthāna, illustrious woman!

39-46: The origin and termination of the nāḍīs.

pūrvabhāge suṣumṇāyā āmeḍhrānte kuhūḥ sthitā |
adhaścordhvaṁ ca kuṇḍalyā vāruṇī sarvagāminī ||39||
yaśasvinī ca yāmyasthā pādāṅguṣṭhāntamiṣyate |
piṅgalā cordhvagā yāmye nāsāntaṁ viddhi me priye ||40||
yāmye pūṣā ca netrāntaṁ piṅgalāyāstu pṛṣṭhataḥ |

[27] Time is a creation of the mind. The flow of prāṇa into iḍā and piṅgalā represent a scattered, dispersed mind. Prāṇa remaining within the suṣumnā represents samādhi—a state of absorption of mind where the perception of time ceases. Therefore, the suṣumnā is described as engulfing time or being beyond time.

payasvinī tathā gārgi yāmyakarṇāntimiṣyate ||41||
sarasvatī tathā cordhvamājihvāyāḥ pratiṣṭhitā |
āsavyakarṇādviprendre śaṅkhinī cordhvagā matā ||42||
gāndhārī savyanetrāntamiḍāyāḥ pṛṣṭhataḥ sthitā |
iḍā ca savyanāsāntaṁ savyabhāge vyavasthitā ||43||
hastijihvā tathā savyapādāṅguṣṭhāntamiṣyate |
viṣvodarā tu yā nāḍī tundamadhye vyavasthitā ||44||
alambuṣā mahābhāge pāyumūlādadhogatā |
etāstvanyāḥ samutpannāḥ śirāścānyāśca tāsvapi ||45||
yathāśvatthadale tadvadabjapatreṣu vā śirāḥ |
nāḍīṣvetāsu sarvāsu vijñātavyāstapodhane ||46||

Kuhu is present in the front region of the suṣumnā, up to the end of the generative organ.

Vāruṇī which spreads everywhere is above and below the kuṇḍalinī.

Yaśasvinī is considered to be on the right side up to the tip of the big toe.

Know that piṅgalā goes upwards up to the nose on the right side, my beloved!

Pūṣā extends on the right up to the eye, at the back of the piṅgalā. Payasvinī is considered to extend up to the right ear, Gārgī!

Sarasvatī is situated upwards, up to the tongue, [Gargi,] illustrious among women!

Śankhinī is said to go upwards up to the left ear.

Gāndhārī extends up to the left eye and is situated behind iḍā. Iḍā is present in the left side, up to the tip of the left nose.

Hastijihvā is said to extend down to the tip of the big toe of the left foot.

The nāḍī visvodarā is situated in the middle of the belly, fortunate [Gārgī]! Alambuṣā goes downwards to the base of the anus region.

The above said nāḍīs and the various other channels that originate from them are similar to the [pattern of the] veins on the leaf of a bodhi tree or a lotus plant. All these nāḍīs and the interconnecting channels are to be known, [Gārgī], rich in austerity!

47-49: The ten vāyus—prāṇa to dhananjaya.

prāṇo'pānaḥsamānaśca udāno vyāna eva ca|
nāgaḥ kūrmo'tha kṛkaro devadatto dhanañjayaḥ ||47||
ete nāḍīṣu sarvāsu caranti daśa vāyavaḥ |
eteṣu vāyavaḥ pañca mukhyāḥ prāṇādayaḥ smṛtāḥ ||48||
teṣu mukhyatamāvetau prāṇāpānau narottame |
prāṇa evatayormukhyaḥ sarvaprāṇabhṛtāṁ sadā ||49||

Prāṇa, apāna, samāna, udāna, vyāna, nāga, kūrma, kṛkara, devadatta, dhananjaya. These ten vāyus (life forces) flow in all these [above said] nāḍīs

Among these, the five vāyus, beginning with prāṇa are considered important. Among those [five vāyus], these two—prāṇa and apāna—are most important, [Gārgī], best among women! And of these two, prāṇa alone is [most] important, in all living beings, always.

50-51: The abode of prāṇa.

āsyanāsikayormadhye hṛnmadhye nābhimadhyame |
prāṇālaya iti prāhuḥ pādāṅguṣṭe'pi kecana ||50||
adhaścordhvaṁ ca kuṇḍalyāḥ parītaḥ prāṇasaṁjñakaḥ |
tiṣṭhanneteṣu sarveṣu prakāśayati dīpavat ||51||

Between the nose and the mouth, in the center of the hṛdaya (heart), in the center of the navel, and by some in the big toe—[this] is said to be the abode of the prāṇa. Present below and above, surrounding the kuṇḍalinī, this one (vāyu) known as prāṇa illuminates the rest of them like a lamp.

52-53: The abode of apāna.

apānanilayaṁ kecid gudameḍhrorujānuṣu |
udare vṛṣaṇe kaṭyāṁ jaṅghe nābhau vadanti hi ||52||
gudāgnyāgārayostiṣṭhanmadhye'pānaḥ prabhañjanaḥ |

adhaścordhvaṁ ca kuṇḍalyāḥ prakāśayati dīpavat ||53||

Some say that the abode of the apāna is in the anus, generative organ, thighs, knees, stomach, testicles, hip, the shanks and in the navel. Situated between the anus and the abode of the fire, the apāna vāyu glows above and below the kuṇḍalinī like a lamp.

54: The abode of vyāna.

vyānaḥ śrotrākṣimadhye ca kṛkaṭyāṁ gulphayorapi |
ghrāṇe gale sphijordeśe tiṣṭhatyatra na saṁśayaḥ ||54||

There is no doubt that vyāna is situated in the center of the ears and the eyes, in the sides of the neck, in the ankles, nose, throat, and posterior region.

55: The abode of udāna.

udānaḥ sarvasandhisthaḥ pādayorhastayorapi |

Udāna is present in all joints, in both legs and the hands as well.

55-57: The abode of samāna.

samānaḥ sarvagātreṣu sarva vyāpya vyavasthitaḥ ||55||
bhuktaṁ sarvarasaṁ gātre vyāpayanvahninā saha |
dvisaptatisahasreṣu nāḍīmargeṣu sañcaret ||56||
samānavāyurevaikaḥ sāgnirvyāpya vyavasthitaḥ |
agnibhiḥ saha sarvatra sāṅgopāṅgakalevare ||57||

The samāna is present in the whole body, spreading everywhere, distributing in the body the essence of what is eaten, along with the fire, it moves in the seventy-two thousand pathways of the nāḍīs. Only the samāna vāyu is present with the fire, along with which it pervades the whole of the body with all its limbs.

58: The abode of the other five vāyus.

nāgādi vāyavaḥ pañca tvagasthyādiṣu saṁsthitāḥ |

The five vāyus starting with nāga are present in the skin, bones etc.

58-66: The process of digestion and assimilation of food and the role of the vāyus in this process.

tundasthaṁ jalamannaṁ ca rasāni ca samīkṛtam ||58||
tundamadhyagataḥ prāṇastāni kuryātpṛthakpṛthak |
punaragnau jalaṁ sthāpya tvannādīni jalopari ||59||
svayaṁ hyapānaṁ saṁprāpya tenaiva saha mārutaḥ |
pravāti jvalanaṁ tatra dehamadhyagataṁ punaḥ ||60||
vāyunā vātito vahnirapānena śanaiḥ śanaiḥ |
tadā jvalati viprendre svakule dehamadhyame ||61||
jvālābhirjvalanastatra prāṇena preritastataḥ |
jalamatyuṣṇamakarotkoṣṭamadhyagataṁ tadā ||62||
annaṁ vyañjanasaṁyuktaṁ jalopari samarpitam |
tataḥ supakvamakarodvahniḥ santaptavāriṇā ||63||
svedamūtre jalaṁ syātāṁ vīryarūpaṁ raso bhavet |
pūrīṣamannaṁ syādgārgi prāṇaḥ kuryātpṛthakpṛthak ||64||
samānavāyunā sārdhaṁ rasaṁ sarvāsu nāḍīṣu |
vyāpayañcchvāsarūpeṇa dehe carati mārutaḥ ||65||
vyomarandhaisca navabhiḥ viṇmūtrādivisarjanam |
kurvanti vāyavaḥ sarve śarīreṣu nirantaram ||66||

The prāṇa in the middle of the belly separates the water, food, and its essence which are [mixed] together in the belly. Then, placing the water in the fire and the food on the water, [the prāṇa] itself becoming (joining) the apāna, along with it, this vāyu kindles the fire in the dehamadhya. The fire fanned slowly by the prāṇa vāyu then burns in its own abode—the dehamadhya, [Gārgī], illustrious among women!

There the fire, its flames kindled by the prāṇa, makes the water in the middle of the belly very hot. The fire through the heated water, cooks the food along with the other ingested ingredients, that have been placed on the water.

The prāṇa converts the water into sweat and urine, the essence of the food (rasa) becomes semen (śukra), and the solid waste is excreted in the form of feces, Gārgī!

The prāṇa, along with the samāna vāyu, spreading the rasa in all the nāḍīs, flows in the body in the form of breath.

The vāyus continuously undertake excretion of waste products, urine etc., in the entire body, through the roots of the hairs and the nine openings.

67-71: The function of each vāyu.

niḥśvāsocchvāsakāsāśca prāṇakarmeti kīrtyate |
apānavāyoḥ karmaitadviṇmūtrādivisarjanam ||67||
hānopādānaceṣṭādi vyānakarmeti ceṣyate |
udānakarma tatproktaṁ dehasyonnayanādi yat ||68||
poṣaṇādi samānasya śarīre karma kīrtitam |
udgārādi guṇo yastu nāgakarmeti kīrtyate ||69||
nimīlanādi kūrmasya kṣutaṁ vai kṛkarasya ca |
devadattasya viprendre tandrīkarmeti kīrtitam ||70||
dhanañjayasya śophādi sarvaṁ karma prakīrtitam |

Inhalation, exhalation, coughing are said to be the functions of the prāṇa.

Excretion of urine, feces etc. is the function of the apāna vāyu.

Actions such as taking, giving are considered as functions of vyāna.

Raising of the body etc. are said to be functions of udāna.

Nutrition is said to be the function of samāna in the body.

Belching etc. are said to be functions of nāga. Blinking, closing of the eyes etc. is kūrma's function, sneezing is kṛkara's and drowsiness is said to be the function of devadatta, illustrious among women! Swelling etc. are all said to be the function of dhanañjaya.

71-72: Instruction to Gārgī to perform nāḍīśodhana.

jñātvaivaṁ nāḍīsaṁsthānaṁ vāyūnāṁ sthānakarmaṇī ||71||
vidhinoktena mārgeṇa nāḍīsaṁśodhanaṁ kuru ||72||
iti śrī yogayājñavalkye caturtho'dhyāyaḥ |

Chapter IV

After thus knowing the position of the nāḍīs and the position and function of the vāyus, undertake the purification of the nāḍīs in the prescribed manner.

The Ten Vayus: Name, Location, Function

Vāyu	Location	Functions
1. Prāṇa	Between nose and jaws, center of the heart, center of navel, big toe, surrounding kuṇḍalinī.	Inhalation, exhalation, coughing, sneezing etc. Separates food, rasa etc.
2. Apāna	Anus, generative organ, thighs, knees, stomach, testicles, kneecap, hip, navel.	Excretion.
3. Vyāna	Between the ear and eyes, sides of the neck, ankles, nose throat, posterior region.	Taking in and giving out.
4. Udāna	All joints, in legs and hands also.	Rising, bending etc.
5. Samāna	Whole body.	Nutrition and growth of the body.
6. Nāga	....	Belching, vomiting etc.
7. Kūrma	....	Opening and closing of the eyes.
8. Kṛkara	....	Sneezing.
9. Devadatta	....	Drowsiness, sleepiness.
10. Dhanañjaya	....	Swelling etc.

*some of these locations and functions differ with ayurvedic texts.

The Fourteen Nāḍīs: Name, Position, Region

Name of the nāḍī	**Position of the nāḍī**	**Region of the nāḍī**
1. Suṣumnā	In the middle of the kandasthāna	Extends up to the top of the head.
2. Iḍā	On the left of the suṣumnā	Extends up to the tip of the left nose on the left side.
3. Piṅgalā	On the right of the suṣumnā	Extends up to the tip of the nose on the right side.
4. Sarasvatī	On the side of the suṣumnā	Extends upwards up to the tongue.
5. Kuhu	On the side of the suṣumnā	From the front region of the suṣumnā up to the end of the generative organ.
6. Gāndhārī	Back of iḍā	Extends up to the left eye.
7. Hastijihvā	Side of iḍā	Extends up to the tip of the big toe of the left foot.
8. Viśvodara	Between kuhu and hastijihvā	In the middle of the the belly.
9. Vāruṇī	Between yaśasvinī and kuhu	Spreads everywhere and is above and below the kunḍalinī.
10. Yaśasvinī	....	Extends on the right side up to the tip of the toe.

Name of the nāḍī	Position of the nāḍī	Region of the nāḍī
11. Payasvinī	Between pūṣā and sarasvatī	Extends up to the right ear.
12. Pūṣā	At the back of the piṅgalā	Extends on the right up to the eye.
13. Śankhinī	Between gāndhārī and sarasvatī	Extends upwards up to the left ear.
14. Alambuṣā	Below the center of the kandasthāna	Extends downwards to the bottom of the anus region.

Chapter V

OUTLINE

1-2: Gārgī's request and Yājñavalkya's assent to teach the method of purification of the nāḍīs.

3-9: The qualities of the aspirant, pre-requisites, ideal environment and daily routine for the practice of yoga.

10-17: The view of some other sages on the environment, lifestyle, and procedure of practice.

17-20: The technique of nāḍīśodhana and duration of practice.

21-22: Results of this practice.

Chapter V

1-2: Gārgī's request and Yājñavalkya's assent to teach the method of purification of the nāḍīs.

gārgyuvāca--
bhagavanbrahmavicchreṣṭha sarvaśāstraviśārada |
kenopayena śuddhāḥ syurnāḍayo me tvaṁ vada prabho ||1||
ityukto brahmavādinyā brahmavidbrāhmaṇastadā |
taṁ samālokya kṛpayā nāḍīśuddhimabhāṣata ||2||

Gārgī said, "One who is fit to be worshipped, the greatest among the ones who have realized the Brahman, master of all the śāstras, please explain to me the method by which the nāḍīs should be purified."

Thus asked by [Gārgī] who seeks the Brahman, [Yājñavalkya] who has realized the highest, looked upon her with compassion and spoke about [the method for] the purification of the nāḍīs.

3-9: The qualities of the aspirant, pre-requisites, ideal environment and daily routine for the practice of yoga.

yājñavalkya uvaca--
vidhyuktakarmasaṁyuktaḥ kāmasaṅkalpavarjitaḥ |
yamaiśca niyamairyuktaḥ sarvasaṅgavivarjitaḥ ||3||
kṛtavidyo jitakrodhaḥ satyadharmaparāyaṇaḥ |
guruśuśruṣaṇarataḥ pitṛmātṛparāyaṇaḥ ||4||
svāśramasthaḥ sadācāraḥ vidvadbhiśca suśikṣitaḥ |
tapovanaṁ susamprāpya phalamūlodakānvitam ||5||
tatra ramye śucau deśe brahmaghoṣasamanvite |
svadharmaniratаiḥ śāntairbrahmavidbhiḥ samāvṛte ||6||
vāribhiśca susampūrṇe puṣpairnānāvidhairyute |
phalamūlaiśca sampūrṇe sarvakāmaphalaprade ||7||
devālaye vā nadyāṁ vā grāme vā nagare'thavā |
suśobhanaṁ maṭhaṁ kṛtvā sarvarakṣāsamanvitam ||8||
trikālasnānasaṁyuktaḥ svadharmanirataḥ sadā |

vedāntaśravaṇaṁ kurvaṁstasminyogaṁ samabhyaset ||9||

Yājñavalkya said:

One who performs all the actions advocated by the Vedas,[28] devoid of desire, endowed with all the yamas and niyamas,[29] uninvolved in worldly affairs, having completed studies [of the śāstras or philosophical treatises], and overcome anger, devoted to adhering to duty and truth, dutifully serves his Guru,[30] devoted to his parents, adhering to [the duties of] his stage in life (āśrama) according to varṇāśramadharma, of good conduct [and character], well educated by great scholars, going to a grove suitable for spiritual pursuits abundant in fruits, roots and good water, in that pleasing pure place which resounds with the chanting of the Vedas, surrounded by tranquil Vedic scholars devoted to their duty, who have realised the Brahman, having built a beautiful, well-protected maṭha[31] near a temple or a flowing river, in a village or a city,[32] abounding in water, filled with fruit and roots, and with flowers of different varieties, the entire surroundings

---

28 Yājñavalkya once again emphasizes the necessity to abide by the Vedas and follow the path of yoga. This is repeated in all the chapters.

29 The ten yamas and the ten niyamas were discussed in detail in Chapters I and II.

30 Serving the guru or teacher is considered an important prerequisite and is also mentioned in the Bhagavad Gita (IV.34).

31 Traditionally, a maṭha was considered a safe place, for the king of the land typically provided complete protection. For example, see the many references to Rama's kingly protection of various sages and their maṭha in the Ramayana.

32 Similar descriptions can be found in the Haṭhayogapradīpikā. For example, Chapter I, verses 12-14 read: "The maṭha should be established in a well-governed prosperous kingdom ruled by a righteous king. The place should be unaffected by water, fire or rocks to the extent of a bow's length. (The measure of a bow's length referred to here is the span of the arms stretched out width wise. This amount of space spherically is sufficient to do the yoga practices.) The place should be free from disturbances and in solitude."

The actual construction of the maṭha has also been explained: "The maṭha should not be too high or too low. It should have a small door and no holes. It should be free from insects and clean, smeared with cow dung. The appearance should be attractive with a hall, a raised seat, a well and a surrounding wall."

capable of bestowing all desired results, [in that maṭha,] the aspirant should bathe thrice a day,[33] always be devoted to his duty, listen to vedānta[34] and practice the path of yoga.

10-17: The view of some other sages on the environment, lifestyle, and procedure of practice.

kecidvadanti munayastapaḥsvādhyāyasaṁyutāḥ |
svadharmaniratāḥ śāntāstantreṣu ca sadā ratāḥ ||10||
nirjane nilaye ramye vātātapavivarjite |
vidhyuktakarmasaṁyuktaḥ śucirbhūtvā samāhitaḥ ||11||
mantrairnyastatanurdhīraḥ sitabhasmadharaḥ sadā |
mṛdvāsanopari kuśānsamāstīrya tato'jinam ||12||
vināyakaṁ susampūjya phalamūlodakādibhiḥ |
iṣṭadevaṁ guruṁ natvā tata āruhya cāsanam ||13||
prāṅmukhodaṅmukho vāpi jitāsanagataḥ svayam |
samagrīvaśiraḥkāyaḥ saṁvṛtāsyaḥ suniścalaḥ ||14||
nāsāgradṛk sadā samyak savye nyasyetaraṁ karam |
nāsāgre śaśabhṛdbimbaṁ jyotsnājālavitānitam ||15||
saptamasya tu vargasya caturthaṁ bindusaṁyutam |
sravantamamṛtaṁ paśyannetrābhyāṁ susamāhitaḥ ||16||

Some sages, endowed with austerity (tapas)[35] and self-study (svādhyāya),[36] devoted to their spiritual duties, peaceful, absorbed in the study of the

---

[33] This does not refer to mere bathing, but means that the daily rituals including meditation and prāṇāyāma should be practiced three times every day.

[34] Anta means "end." Thus, vedānta means "the end (essence) of the Vedas." The Vedas have four parts: samhitā, brāhmaṇa, āraṇyaka, and upaniṣad. The last part (the end) of the Vedas, the upaniṣad, are considered the vedānta. The essence of the upaniṣads has been presented in the form of the Brahmasūtra by Vyāsa. The Brahmasūtra is also referred to as vedānta.

[35] The root of the word, tapas, is "tap" meaning "to burn." In this context, "burning" refers to reduction of impurities of the body and the mind (kleśas).

[36] Svādhyāya: the word can be split and understood as sva, "self," adhi, "near," and ayana, "to go." The effort of moving closer to one's true self is svādhyāya.

tantras say, "In an uninhabited pleasant abode, without [excessive] heat or wind, performing the deeds said in the Vedas, after becoming pure and focused, the aspirant who is strong and persevering, with a body controlled with the help of mantras, always wearing the white sacred ash,[37] laying down tender special grass and deer skin, having worshipped Vināyaka (or Ganeśa, the remover of obstacles), with fruits, roots etc., after saluting his personal deity and guru, then ascending the seat facing east or north, assuming a comfortable and steady posture, keeping his neck, head and body erect in alignment, with his mouth closed, remaining steady (without any movement), placing his right hand on his left [hand], steadying his gaze well on the tip of his nose[38] always, focusing on the moon with its cool rays, with the flow of nectar from the tip of the head representing the tūrīya avasthā."[39]

17-20: The technique of nāḍīśodhana and duration of practice.

iḍayā vāyumāropya pūrayitvodarasthitam |
tato'gniṁ dehamadhyasthaṁ dhyāyanjvālāvalīyutam ||17||
rephaṁ ca bindusaṁyuktamagnimaṇḍalasaṁsthitam |
dhyāyanvirecayetpaścānmandaṁ piṅgalayā punaḥ ||18||
punaḥ piṅgalayāpūrya prāṇaṁ dakṣiṇataḥ sudhīḥ |

---

[37] The daily rituals prescribed in the Vedas involve worshipping the Divine using fire. The ashes left after performing these ceremonies are the "sacred ashes" referred to here, and are smeared on the body. This is also mentioned in Chapter I.

[38] A very similar procedure is detailed in the Bhagavad Gita (VI.13-17). The aspirant should be free from desire for fruits of actions, free of motivations, should have control over himself and be in solitude. The seat for the practice should be prepared with kuśa grass, deerskin, and a cloth, situated in a clean place, firmly fixed, neither too high nor too low. Sitting on that seat, he should focus his mind totally, having controlled the senses and practice yoga. He should hold his body, neck and head still and upright, focusing his gaze on the tip of his nose, without distraction. He should be tranquil and, fearless, and controlling his mind, should meditate upon the Divine.

[39] Tūrīya avasthā is usually understood as the fourth state of consciousness, beyond the three normal states of waking, deep sleep, and dreaming.

punarvirecayeddhīmāniḍayā tu śanaiḥ śanaiḥ ||19||
tricaturvatsaraṁ vātha tricaturmāsameva vā |
ṣaṭkṛtva ācarennityaṁ rahasyevaṁ trisandhiṣu ||20||

Having inhaled the air through the left nostril filling up [the chest and abdomen], then meditating on the fire in the belly with its flames in the dehamadhya and meditating on the seed letter of fire ("ram") established in the region of fire he must exhale afterwards slowly through the right nostril.

Then the determined and wise [practitioner], inhaling the air through the right nostril, must again exhale slowly through the left nostril.[40] One should practice this in solitude six times everyday in the morning, afternoon, and evening for three to four months or three to four years.

21-22: Results of this practice.

nāḍīśuddhimavāpnoti pṛthak cihnopalakṣitām |
śarīralaghutā dīptirvahnerjaṭharavartinaḥ ||21||
nādābhivyaktirityete cihnaṁ tatsiddhisūcakam |
yāvadetāni sampaśyettāvadeva samācaret ||22||
iti śrīyogayājñavalkye pañcamo'dhyāyaḥ |

One attains nāḍīśuddhi (purity of the nāḍīs), indicated by certain characteristics: lightness of the body, enhancement of the metabolic fire (jaṭharāgni) improvement in the voice (nāda).[41]

These changes are indicative of its attainment (of the nāḍīs being purified). One should continue to practice thus until these [above mentioned changes] are experienced.

---

[40] One nostril should be fully closed, and the other partially closed if possible, to facilitate subtle and long exhalation and inhalation.

[41] The Haṭhayogapradīpikā (II.19-20) also describes similar benefits. When the nāḍīs are cleansed, certain changes can be observed, including lightness and luster in the body, control over the breath, enhanced agni (digestion or metabolism), and improvement in one's voice.

Chapter VI

OUTLINE

1: Yājñavalkya begins his discourse on prāṇāyāma.

2-3: Definition of prāṇāyāma.

4-7: One type of prāṇāyāma.

8-10: Another type of prāṇāyāma.

11-15: Mantras to be used by a brahmin during prāṇāyāma.

16-23: Mantras to be used by others and the benefits of such a prāṇāyāma practice.

24-25: Definition of inhalation, holding, and exhalation.

26-35: The three grades of prāṇāyāma. Explanation of kevala kumbhaka and sahita kumbhaka, and the benefits thereof.

36-38: The method to attain mastery over the prāṇa and the benefits of such mastery.

39-49: Benefits of focusing the prāṇa at various places in the body.

50-53: Another means to master the prāṇa (ṣaṇmukhī mudrā).

54-58: Prāṇāyāma and nāda.

59-64: Another means to master the prāṇa (an alternative to the ṣaṇmukhī mudrā). The mantras to be used by the four divisions during the practice.

65-75: Prāṇāyāma and kuṇḍalinī: burning and awakening of the kuṇḍalinī and the ascent of the prāṇa to the brahmarandhra.

76-78: Prāṇāyāma practice for union with the Divine.

79-82: The virtues of prāṇāyāma and the importance of its practice.

Chapter VI

1: Yājñavalkya begins his discourse on prāṇāyāma.

yājñavalkya uvāca--
prāṇāyāmathādīnāṁ pravakṣyāmi vidhānataḥ |
samāhitamanāstvaṁ ca śṛṇu gārgi varānane ||1||

Yājñavalkya said, "Now,[42] I am now going to speak about prāṇāyāma in an orderly manner. Beautiful Gārgī, listen to me with a focused mind."

2-3: Definition of prāṇāyāma.

prāṇāpānasamāyogaḥ prāṇāyāma itīritaḥ |
prāṇāyāma iti prokto recakapūrakakumbhakaiḥ ||2||
varṇatrayātmakā hyete recakapūrakakumbhakāḥ |
sa eṣa praṇavaḥ proktaḥ prāṇāyāmaśca tanmayaḥ ||3||

Balancing prāṇa and apāna is said to be prāṇāyāma. Prāṇāyāma is said to

---

[42] Many Vedic texts begin with the Sanskrit word, "atha," which is commonly translated as "now." For example, the Yogasūtra begin with "atha yogānuśāsanam" and the Brahmasutras begin with "athātho brahmajijñāsā." This word is considered to be auspicious, since "atha" and "OM" are said to have originated from the throat of Brahmā, the creator. "Now" in this context, means "now the student is ready to receive the teachings." It means that the student has fulfilled the requirements laid out in the previous chapters, as below:

Adherence to the yamas and niyamas (Chapters I and II).

Mastery of the āsana for the practice of prāṇāyāma (Chapter III). (In the Yogasūtra, Vyasa in his commentary on II.49, the sutra on prāṇāyāma, expresses the same opinion. He says "sati āsana jaye" which means "Having mastered āsana..." Note, however, that no specific posture is indicated.)

Clear knowledge of the position of the nāḍīs, the vāyus, and their functions (Chapter IV).

Attainment of purity of the nāḍīs (Chapter V).

consist of exhale (recaka), inhale (pūraka) and holding (kumbhaka).[43] These three components of prāṇāyāma namely exhale, inhale and holding are of the nature of three syllables (A, U, M). [Thereby] prāṇāyāma is of the form of the praṇava (the mantra "OM").[44]

4-7: One type of prāṇāyāma.

iḍayā vāyumāropya pūrayitvodarasthitam |
śanaiḥ ṣoḍaśabhirmātrairakāraṁ tatra saṁsmaret ||4||
dhārayet pūritaṁ paścāccatuḥṣaṣṭhyā tu mātrayā |
ukāramūrtimatrāpi saṁsmaranpraṇavaṁ japet ||5||
yāvadvā śakyate tāvaddhāraṇaṁ japasaṁyutam |
pūritaṁ recayet paścātprāṇaṁ bāhyānilānvitam ||6||
śanaiḥ piṅgalayā gārgi dvātriṁśanmātrayā punaḥ |
makāramūrtimatrāpi saṁsmaranpraṇavaṁ japet ||7||

Inhaling the air slowly for sixteen units (matras) through the left nostril, filling the belly (chest and abdomen) one must meditate on [the deity represented by] "A".[45] Then one must retain the inhaled air for sixty four units thinking of [the deity represented by] "U" and meditate on the praṇava. Otherwise, retain the breath for as long as possible, with

---

[43] The order in which the three components are mentioned here is significant: recaka (exhale), pūraka (inhale), and kumbhaka (holding). This same order is specified in the Yogasūtra (II.50), and indicated in the Bhagavad Gita (IV.29).

[44] Equating prāṇāyāma with OM has a basis in the connection between the microcosm and macrocosm. In the microcosm, prāṇa is the life force and the basis for all creation, sustenance, and destruction in the body. Likewise in the macrocosm, OM represents the Divine and the three letters of OM—A, U, and M—symbolize creation, sustenance, and destruction, respectively. Prāṇāyāma will later be defined with the gāyatrī mantra, which can be used to measure the length of inhale, exhale, and hold. The use of gāyatrī with prāṇāyāma is described in verses 4-10 from the alternate recension at the end of this chapter.

[45] Various bhāvanas are possible during the practice. According to one of these interpretations, A represents Viṣṇu or God, U represents Lakṣmī or the Mother Goddess, and M represents the self (jīva). In this representation, U, the Mother Goddess, can be thought of as the link between the self (M) and the Divine (A).

repetition of the mantra (japa). Then exhale slowly[46] the inhaled air for thirty-two units to join the air outside through the right nostril (piṅgalā). Here too, thinking of [the deity represented by] "M," meditate on the praṇava, Gārgī.

8-10: Another type of prāṇāyāma.

prāṇāyāmo bhavedeṣaḥ punaścaīvaṁ samabhyaset |
tataḥ piṅgalayāpūrya mātraiḥ ṣoḍaśabhistathā ||8||
ukāramūrtimatrāpi saṁsmaransusamāhitaḥ |
pūritaṁ dhārayetprāṇaṁ praṇavaṁ viṁśatidvayam ||9||
japedatra smaranmūrtiṁ makārākhyaṁ maheśvaram |
yāvadvā śakyate paścādrecayediḍayānilam ||10||

This is prāṇāyāma. One must do this again (repeatedly). Inhaling through the right nostril for sixteen units thinking of [the deity represented by] "U" here too, with a focused mind, one must hold the inhaled air, thinking of "M" representing Maheśvara[47] repeating forty times or for as long as possible, and then one must exhale the air through the left nostril.

11-15: Mantras to be used by a brahmin during prāṇāyāma.

evameva punaḥ kuryādiḍayāpūrya pūrvavat |
nāḍyā prāṇaṁ samāropya pūrayitvodarasthitam ||11||
praṇavena susaṁyuktāṁ vyāhṛtībhiśca saṁyutām |
gāyatrīṁ ca japedvipraḥ prāṇasamyamane trayaḥ ||12||

---

[46] The practitioner must first master slow and smooth exhalation. Thus many texts say that exhale should not be fast. For example, the HYP (II.9) says, "exhale slowly, not fast." Holding the breath should not affect the quality of the exhalation.

[47] The word "Brahman" is of neuter gender. One can relate to it as either masculine or feminine. Various mental attitudes may be used during the practice of prāṇāyāma. This manuscript refers to Maheśvara ("Supreme God"), while yet another version refers to Maheśvarī ("Supreme Goddess"), who is the mother of the universe. However, as already mentioned, the masculine and feminine aspects are considered to be inseparable.

punaścaivaṁ tribhiḥ kuryātpunaścaiva trisandhiṣu |
yadvā samabhyasennityaṁ vaidikaṁ laukikaṁ tu vā ||13||
prāṇasaṁyamane vidvānjapettadviṁśatidvayam |
brāhmaṇaḥ śrutasampannaḥ svadharmaniratah sadā ||14||
sa vaidikaṁ japenmantraṁ laukikaṁ na kadācana |
kecidbhūtahitārthāya japamicchanti laukikam ||15||

One must do this again (repeatedly). Inhaling as before through the left nostril, taking the air in, having filled the [chest and] abdomen, a brahmin should repeat the gāyatrī mantra three times accompanied by OM and the vyāhrtis[48] during prāṇāyāma.

One must do this three times in the morning, afternoon and evening. Or, the learned one should, everyday, during prāṇāyāma, do forty repetitions of mantras, Vedic or laukika.[49]

A brahmin who has studied the Vedas, who is devoted to the performance of his duty, should always do meditation with only Vedic mantras, never laukika mantras. There are some who consider that meditation (japa) with laukika mantras can be done for the welfare of living beings.

16-23: Mantras to be used by others and the benefits of such a prāṇāyāma practice.

dvijavatkṣātrasyoktaḥ prāṇasaṁyamane japaḥ |
vaiśyānāṁ dharmayuktānāṁ strīśūdrāṇāṁ tapasvinām ||16||
prāṇasaṁyamane gārgi mantraṁ praṇavavarjitam |
namontaṁ śivamantraṁ vā vaiṣṇavaṁ veṣyate budhaiḥ ||17||
yadvā samabhyasecchūdro laukikaṁ vidhipūrvakam |
prāṇasaṁyamane strī ca japettadviṁśatidvayam ||18||

---

[48] The vyahṛtis here refer to the words "bhūḥ bhuvaḥ suvaḥ" found in the gāyatrī mantra.

[49] A mantra used to gain spiritual progress or stillness of the mind (jñāna) is vaidika. A mantra used to gain worldly benefits is laukika.

na vaidikaṁ japecchūdraḥ striyaśca na kadācana |
svāśramasthasya vaiśyasya kecidicchanti vaidikam ||19||
sandhyayorubhayornityaṁ gāyatryā praṇavena vā |
prāṇasaṁyamanaṁ kuryāt brāhmaṇo vedapāragaḥ ||20||
nityameva prakurvīta prāṇāyāmāṁstu ṣoḍaśa |
api bhrūṇahanaṁ māsātpunantyaharahaḥ kṛtāḥ ||21||
ṛtutrayātpunantyenaṁ janmāntarakṛtādaghāt |
vatsarādbrahmahā śuddhyettasmānnityaṁ samabhyaset ||22||
yogābhyāsaratāstvevaṁ svadharmaniratāśca ye |
prāṇasaṁyamanenaiva sarve muktā bhavanti hi ||23||

Japa during prāṇāyāma is said for kṣatriyas to be the same as for brahmins. For vaiśyas, women and the fourth division who are of good conduct (dharma) and practicing austerity (tapas), during prāṇāyāma, mantras without the praṇava, ending with namaḥ,[50] relating to Śiva or Viṣṇu are recommended by the wise. Otherwise, women and the fourth division must meditate with laukika mantras (mantras other than from the Vedas), forty times in the proper manner, during [the practice of] prāṇāyāma. Women and the fourth division are not to do meditation with vaidika mantras. Some say that vaiśyas who follow the duties of their āśrama can use Vedic mantras.

A brahmin who has mastered the Vedas must do prāṇāyāma with the gāyatrī mantra or praṇava every morning and evening. One must always practice prāṇāyāma thus sixteen times.

Done [day after day] for a month, [prāṇāyāma] purifies even one who has committed [the crime of] abortion. In six months, it purifies the sins of earlier births. In a year even one who had killed a brahmin will be

---

[50] The word, "namaḥ" signifies surrender. "Na" means "not" and "maḥ" means "mine." Thus "namaḥ" means "not mine." Many mantras begin or end with namaḥ, for example "śivāya namaḥ" (surrender to the deity Śiva) or Viṣṇave namaḥ (surrendering to the deity Viṣṇu).

purified.[51] Those who are devoted to their dharma and the practice of yoga, will all be freed through [the practice of] prāṇāyāma itself. Therefore one must practice [prāṇāyāma] everyday.

24-25: Definition of inhalation, holding, and exhalation.

bāhyādāpūraṇaṁ vāyorudare pūrako hi saḥ |
sampūrṇakumbhavadvāyordhāraṇaṁ kumbhako bhavet ||24||
bahiryadrecanaṁ vāyorudarādrecakaḥ smṛtaḥ |

Taking in the air from outside and filling the [chest and] abdomen is inhale, retaining the air [in the chest and abdomen] like a filled pot is retention. Expelling the air out from the [chest and] abdomen is called exhale.

26-35: The three grades of prāṇāyāma. Explanation of kevala kumbhaka and sahita kumbhaka, and the benefits thereof.

prasvedajanako yastu prāṇāyāmeṣu so'dhamaḥ ||25||
kampako madhyamaḥ prokta utthānaścottamo bhavet |
pūrvaṁ pūrvaṁ prakurvīta yāvaduttamasambhavaḥ ||26||
sambhavatyuttame gārgi prāṇāyāme sukhī bhavet |
prāṇo layati tenaiva dehasyāntastato'dhikaḥ ||27||
dehaścottiṣṭhate tena kṛtāsanaparigrahaḥ |
niḥśvāsocchvāsakau tasya na vidyete kathaṁcana ||28||
dehe yadyapi tau syātāṁ svābhāvikaguṇāvubhau |
tathāpi naśyatastena prāṇāyāmottamena hi ||29||
tayornāśe samarthaḥ syātkartuṁ kevalakumbhakam |

---

[51] The Vedas are called "śruti," from the root, "śru" meaning "to hear." The Vedas were not written down, but memorized and transmitted orally. The brahmins were the repository of the Vedic knowledge. Therefore, in those days, killing a brahmin was considered a serious offense as it amounted to the destruction of knowledge. In return, the brahmin was expected to lead a transparently simple life, devoted principally to learning, teaching, and spiritual practice. He was expected to shun the chase for wealth and power, and instead be sustained chiefly by the goodwill and respect of the society he served.

recakaṁ pūrakaṁ muktvā sukhaṁ yadvāyudhāraṇam ||30||
prāṇāyāmo'yamityuktaḥ sa vai kevalakumbhakaḥ |
recya cāpūrya yaḥ kuryātsa vai sahitakumbhakaḥ ||31||
sahitaṁ kevalaṁ cātha kumbhakaṁ nityamabhyaset |
yāvatkevalasiddhiḥ syāttāvatsahitamabhyaset ||32||
kevale kumbhake siddhe recapūraṇavarjite |
na tasya durlabhaṁ kiñcittriṣu lokeṣu vidyate||33||
manojavatvaṁ labhate palitādi ca naśyati |
mukterayaṁ mahāmārgo makārākhyāntarātmanaḥ ||34||

That prāṇāyāma which produces excessive perspiration is the lowest among the types of prāṇāyāma. The one which causes trembling [in the body] is said to be average. The one that makes the body [feel light enough to] rise up is the best prāṇāyāma.

Each preceding one (prāṇāyāma) must be done until the best one is attained. When the highest prāṇāyāma is attained, one reaches a state of comfort and joy. The prāṇa that was scattered becomes contained in the body (the suṣumnā) through this prāṇāyāma.[52] The body, firmly seated in āsana, rises by this [prāṇāyāma].

Inhale and exhale do not exist for him anymore. Though they are both qualities inherent in the body, by that highest prāṇāyāma, they perish (subside), nevertheless. When these two [inhale and exhale] subside, one becomes fit to practice kevala kumbhaka.

The prāṇāyāma where the breath is held inside effortlessly, letting go of inhale and exhale, it is said to be kevala kumbhaka. The one (prāṇāyāma) done by inhaling and exhaling is sahita kumbhaka. Sahita kumbhaka and kevala kumbhaka must both be practiced. Sahita kumbhaka must be practiced till kevala kumbhaka is attained completely.

---

[52] The stages of prāṇāyāma are explained similarly in the Haṭhayogapradīpikā (II.12).

When kevala kumbhaka, without inhale and exhale is attained, there is nothing that is unattainable for him (the yogi) in the three worlds. One acquires total control over the mind, and old age vanishes. This path is the highest one leading to the liberation of the self, signified by [the seed letter] "M."

36-38: The method to attain mastery over the prāṇa and the benefits of such mastery.

nādaṁ cotpādayatyeṣaḥ kumbhakaḥ prāṇasaṁyamaḥ |
prāṇasaṁsayanaṁ nāma dehe prāṇasya dhāraṇam ||35||
eṣaḥ prāṇajayopāyaḥ sarvamṛtyūpaghātakaḥ |
kiñcitprāṇajayopāyaṁ tava vakṣyāmi tattvataḥ ||36||
bāhyātprāṇaṁ samākṛṣya pūrayitvodarasthitam |
nābhimadhye ca nāsāgre pādāṅguṣṭhe ca yatnataḥ ||37||
dhārayenmanasā prāṇaṁ sandhyākāleṣu sarvadā |
sarvarogavinirmukto jīvedyogī gataklamaḥ ||38||

Kumbhaka prāṇāyāma causes the appearance of nāda.[53] Retaining the prāṇa within the body is called prāṇāyāma. This method of mastery over the prāṇa (kevala kumbhaka), leads to absence of disease and death.[54]

I will tell you, in the proper manner, one methodology to attain mastery over prāṇa. Having inhaled the air from outside and filled the chest and abdomen, one must endeavour to retain the prāṇa, through the [effort of the] mind, in the navel, tip of the nose and the big toes during the morning, afternoon and evening, always. The yogi [who practices this] lives free from all diseases and fatigue.

---

[53] Nāda is heard when the nāḍīs are cleansed by the practice of prāṇāyāma. Nādānusandhāna is explained in detail in the Haṭhayogapradīpikā (Chapter IV).

[54] Proper practice of prāṇāyāma leads to absence of disease. "Absence of death" means that the person gaines the experience that he is not the body.

39-49: Benefits of focusing the prāṇa at various places in the body.

nāsāgre dhāraṇaṁ gārgi vāyorvijayakāraṇam |
sarvarogavināśaḥ syānnābhimadhye ca dhāraṇāt ||39||
śarīra laghutāṁ yāti pādāṅguṣṭhe ca dhāraṇāt |
rasanāvāyumākṛṣya yaḥ pibetsatataṁ naraḥ ||40||
śramadāhau na tasyāstāṁ naśyanti vyādhayastathā |
sandhyayorbrāhmakāle vā vāyumakṛṣya yaḥ pibet ||41||
trimāsāttasya kalyāṇi jāyate vāksarasvatī |
ṣaṇmāsābhyāsayogena mahārogaiḥ pramucyate ||42||
ātmanyātmānamāropya kuṇḍalyāṁ yastu dhārayet |
kṣayarogādayastasya naśyantītyapare viduḥ ||43||
jihvayā vāyumānīya jihvāmūle nirodhayan |
yaḥ pibedamṛtaṁ vidvānsakalaṁ bhadramaśnute ||44||
ātmanyātmānamiḍayā samānīya bhruvontare |
pibedyastridaśāhāraṁ vyādhibhiḥ sa vimucyate ||45||
nāḍībhyāṁ vāyumāropya nābhau vā tundapārśvayoḥ |
ghaṭikaikāṁ vahedyastu vyādhibhiḥ so'bhimucyate ||46||
māsamekaṁ trisandhyāyāṁ jihvayāropya mārutam |
pibedyastridaśāhāraṁ dhārayettundamadhyame ||47||
gulmāṣṭhīlā plīhā cānye tridoṣajanitāstathā |
tundamadhyagatā rogāḥ sarve naśyanti tasya vai ||48||
jvarāḥ sarve vinaśyanti viṣāṇi vividhāni ca |
bahunoktena kiṁ gārgi palitādi ca naśyati ||49||

Gārgī, focusing [the prāṇa] at the tip of the nose, is the way to master the prāṇa. By focusing on the navel all diseases are removed. The body attains lightness by focusing on the big toes.[55]

---

[55] In explaining the various types of prāṇāyāma to overcome disease and stay healthy, Yājñavalkya emphasizes the effect of bhāvana in prāṇāyāma.

The person who inhales the air through the tongue constantly[56] has no fatigue, and heat and diseases perish. One who inhales air (practices prāṇāyāma) thus in the morning, afternoon and evening or before sunrise (brāhmamuhūrta) for three months acquires proficiency in speech, blessed [Gārgī]. By practising for six months one becomes free of all diseases.

Some others opine that if one turns the mind inward and focuses on the kuṇḍalinī, diseases related to degeneration, decay etc. are destroyed. The learned one who inhales the air through the tongue, retains it at the base of the tongue, and drinks the nectar, attains all benefits.[57]

The one who controls and focuses the mind, inhaling through the left nostril, focusing [on the space] between the eyebrows and drinks nectar is freed from diseases.

One who inhales through both nostrils focusing [the prāṇa] on the navel or either sides of the belly, [and continues the cycle] for twenty-four minutes (holding one minute after inhale for twenty-four times) is quickly relieved from diseases.

For one who inhales through the tongue and drinks the nectar, focusing on the belly, during morning, afternoon, and evening for one month, is freed of all diseases of the spleen, and other diseases. All diseases caused by the three doṣas[58] and diseases of the stomach too are all destroyed. All fevers and various toxins are destroyed. Why say more Gārgī, even old age is destroyed.

50-53: Another means to master the prāṇa (ṣaṇmukhī mudrā).

evaṁ vāyujayopāyaḥ prāṇasya tu varānane |

---

[56] This type of prāṇāyāma is called "śītalī prāṇāyāma." It is praised as being useful in many debilitating diseases (mahārogas).

[57] This prāṇāyāma includes jihvā bandha. Attention focused at the root of the tongue leads to an increased sharpness of the senses.

[58] In ayurveda, the three doṣas are vāta, pitta and kapha.

śakyamāsanamāsthāya samāhitamanāstathā ||50||
karaṇāni vaśīkṛtya viṣayebhyo balātsudhīḥ |
apānamūrdhvamākṛṣya praṇavena samāhitaḥ ||51||
hastābhyāṁ bandhayetsamyakkarṇādi karaṇāni ca |
aṅguṣṭābhyāmubhe śrotre tarjanībhyāṁ ca cakṣuṣī ||52||
nāsāpuṭau madhyamābhyāṁ pracchādya karaṇāni vai |
ānandānubhavaṁ yāvattāvanmūrddhani dhārayet ||53||

Thus is the means for mastery over prāṇa, beautiful [Gārgī]! Assuming a posture one is capable of [staying in], with a focused mind, controlling the senses and drawing them away from their objects, the wise one, pulling the apāna upwards, having controlled the mind using the praṇava (meditating on the praṇava), restrain the ears and the other senses with the hands. Close the two ears with the thumbs, the eyes with the index fingers, and the nostrils with the middle fingers,[59] [and having thus restrained all the senses,] focus on the crown of the head, till the state of bliss (ānanda) is experienced.

54-58: Prāṇāyāma and nāda.

prāṇaḥ prayātyanenaiva tatastvāyurvighātakṛt |
brahmarandhre suṣumṇāyāṁ mṛṇālāntarasūtravat ||54||
nādotpattistvanenaiva śuddhasphaṭikasannibhā |
āmūrdhno vartate nādo vīṇādaṇḍavadutthitaḥ ||55||
śaṁkhadhvaninibhastvādau madhye meghadhvaniryathā |
vyomaranghre gate nāde giriprasravaṇaṁ yathā ||56||
vyomaranghre gate vāyau citte cātmani saṁsthite |
tadānandī bhaveddehī vāyustena jito bhavet ||57||
yoginastvapare hyatra vadanti samacetasaḥ |
prāṇāyāmaparāḥ pūtā recapūraṇavarjitāḥ ||58||

By this practice, the prāṇa which causes reduction of the life span (when it

[59] This is called "ṣaṇmukhī mudrā."

is dispersed), [is centered and] moves into the brahmarandhra, through the suṣumnā nāḍī, like a fiber inside a lotus stalk. The appearance of pure and crystalline nāda (sound), present up to the top of the head like the sound produced by a vīṇā[60] (a traditional musical string instrument), is due to this [movement].

At first, the sound produced by a conch [is heard], then sounds of thunder, and when the nāda reaches the crown of the head (brahmarandhra), a sound similar to a mountain waterfall [is heard].[61] When the prāṇa vāyu reaches the brahmarandhra, and the mind is absorbed in the self, the practitioner becomes blissful and prāṇa is conquered by him. Other yogis who are dedicated to the practice of prāṇāyāma, who are pure, and who have gone beyond inhale and exhale, having similar views on this, also say thus.

59-64: Another means to master the prāṇa (an alternative to the ṣaṇmukhī mudrā). The mantras to be used by the four divisions during the practice.

dakṣiṇetaragulphena sīvanīṁ pīḍayet śirām |
aghastādaṇḍayoḥ sūkṣmāṁ savyopari ca dakṣiṇam ||59||
jaṅghorvorantaraṁ gārgi niśchidraṁ bandhayeddṛḍham |
samagrīvaśiraskandhaḥ samapṛṣṭhaḥ samodaraḥ ||60||
netrābhyāṁ dakṣiṇaṁ gulphaṁ lokayannuparisthitam |
dhārayanmanasā sārdhaṁ vyāharanpraṇavākṣaram ||61||
āsane nānyadhīrāste dvijo rahasi nityaśaḥ |
kṣatriyaśca varārohe vyāharanpraṇavākṣaram ||62||

---

[60] The human spine is comparable to the vīṇā, an ancient Indian string instrument, the vertebrae of the spine being likened to the nodes of the vīṇā. The practice of mūlabandha tightens the base of the spine, similar to the tightening of the vīṇā at its base. Only when the strings are properly tightened and in proper tension, is the sound (nāda) from the vīṇā proper. Similarly, the practice of the bandhas are useful for proper nādānusandhāna .

[61] The fourth chapter of the Haṭhayogapradīpikā deals extensively with nādānusandhāna and the sounds described are similar.

āsane nānyadhīraste rahasyeva jitendriyaḥ |
vaiśyāḥ śūdrāḥ striyaścānye yogābhyāsaratāḥ narāḥ ||63||
śaivaṁ vā vaiṣṇavaṁ vātha vyāharannanyameva vā |
āsane nānyadhīraste dīpaṁ haste vilokayan ||64||

Press the perineum beneath the generative organ by the left ankle and place the right ankle on the left. Close the thighs and the knees together firmly, without a gap in between. A brahmin, keeping the neck, head, shoulders and the back and belly straight, looking with the eyes at the right ankle on top, mentally focusing and reciting the praṇava [extended by half a matra], must sit in āsana, in solitude, without distraction everyday.[62] A kṣatriya must sit in the [above] āsana in solitude everyday without distraction and total focus, repeating the praṇava with complete control over the senses. Vaiśyas, women, the fourth division and others who are keen on practising yoga must sit in āsana repeating mantras on Śiva or Viṣṇu or other mantras without distraction, gazing at a lamp [held] in their hands.

65-75: Prāṇāyāma and kuṇḍalinī: burning and awakening of the kuṇḍalinī and the ascent of the prāṇa to the brahmarandhra.

āyurvighātakṛtprāṇastvanenāgnikulaṁ gataḥ |
dhūmadhvajajayaṁ yāvannānyadhīrevamabhyaset ||65||
dhāraṇaṁ kurvatastasya śaktiḥ syādiṣṭabhojane |
dehaśca laghutāṁ yāti jaṭharāgniśca vardhate ||66||
dṛṣṭacihnastatastasmānmanasāropya mārutam |
mantramuccārayandīrghaṁ nābhimadhye nirodhayet ||67||
yāvanmano layatyasminnābhau savitṛmaṇḍale |
tāvatsamabhyasedvidvānniyato niyatāsanaḥ ||68||
etena nābhimadhyasthadhāraṇenaiva mārutaḥ |
kuṇḍalīṁ yāti vahniśca dahatyatra na saṁśayaḥ ||69||
santaptā vahninā tatra vāyunā cālitā svayam |
prasāryaṁ phaṇabhṛdbhogaṁ prabodhaṁ yāti sā tadā ||70||

---

[62] An alternative to ṣaṇmukhī mudrā is offered here.

prabuddhe saṁsaratyasminnābhimūle tu cakriṇi |
brahmarandhre suṣumṇāyāṁ prayāti prāṇasaṁjñakaḥ ||71||
saṁprāpte mārute tasminsuṣumṇāyāṁ varānane |
mantramuccārya manasā hṛnmadhye dhārayetpunaḥ ||72||
hṛdayātkaṇṭhakūpe ca bhruvormadhye ca dhārayet |
tasmādāropya manasā sāgniṁ prāṇamananyadhīḥ ||73||
dhārayedvyomni viprendre vyāharanpraṇavākṣaram |
vāyunā pūrite vyomni sāṅgopāṅge kalevare ||74||
tadātmā rājate tatra yathā vyomni vikartanaḥ |

By this, prāṇa, which [on being dispersed] reduces the life span, reaches the abode of agni (fire). Until one gains mastery over agni, one must continue to practice thus without any distraction. One who holds [the prāṇa thus] will have the strength to digest whatever is eaten. Jaṭharāgni (metabolic or digestive fire) is enhanced and the body becomes light.

After having experienced the above signs, taking the prāṇa upwards, by the mind, hold it in the middle of the belly for a long time, reciting the mantra. The learned one must sit in the [prescribed] posture properly, with discipline (observing all the prerequisites mentioned earlier) and do the [above] practice till the mind is totally absorbed in the abode of the Divine (savitṛmaṇḍala) in the navel region. By this focus (dhāraṇa) in the navel, the prāṇa reaches the kunḍalinī and the agni burns it (the kunḍalinī). There is no doubt on this.

Burnt by the fire, fanned by the vāyu, she (the kunḍalinī) then, spreads her hood and awakens. When she is awakened, the prāṇa moves in this cakra at the base of the navel (nābhi) and moves in the suṣumnā towards the brahmarandhra.

Beautiful [Gārgī], as the prāṇa reaches (moves through) that suṣumnā, one must recite the mantra mentally and hold it (the prāṇa) again in the center of the heart (hṛdaya).

Then, from the heart, one must hold the prāṇa in the root of the throat and in the point between the eyebrows.

From there one must raise the prāṇa along with the agni, and retain it in the crown of the head (brahmarandhra), while reciting the praṇava (the mantra OM) without distraction.

Gārgī, when the prāṇa pervades the brahmarandhra, the self shines throughout the entire body like the sun in the sky.

76-78: Prāṇāyāma practice for union with the Divine.

śarīraṁ visusṛkṣuścedevaṁ samyak samācaran ||75||
ekākṣaraṁ paraṁ brahma dhyāyanpraṇavamīśvaram |
saṁbhidya manasā mūrdhni brahmarandhraṁ savāyunā ||76||
prāṇamunmocayetpaścānmahāprāṇe khamadhyame |
dehātīte jagatprāṇe śūnye nitye dhruve pade ||77||
ākāśe paramānande svātmānaṁ yojayeddhiyā |
brahmevāsau bhavedgārgi na punarjanmabhāgbhavet ||78||

One who desires to leave the body,[63] then, practicing this (the above said prāṇāyāma) properly, meditating on Divine, the cosmic consciousness, [represented by] the praṇava,[64] opening the brahmarandhra in the crown of the head by the mind along with the prāṇa, must then unite the prāṇa with the mahāprāṇa,[65] which supports the entire world, which is [represented by] space, [existing] beyond attributes, eternal and everlasting.

Unite the self with that space, the ultimate fulfillment (paramānanda), with determination. Such a person becomes one with the Brahman and is not subject to birth again (transcends the cycle of birth and death).

79-82: The virtues of prāṇāyāma and the importance of its practice.

tasmāttvaṁ ca varārohe nityaṁ karma samācāra |

---

[63] Refer also Bhagavad Gita (Chapter 8).

[64] The praṇava is considered a way to address Īśvara, the Divine (refer Yogasūtra I.27).

[65] When the prāṇa is said to join the mahāprāṇa, it should be understood as the Seer (jīvātmā), mounted on the prāṇa, joins the Divine (paramātmā).

sandhyākāleṣu vā nityaṁ prāṇasaṁyamanaṁ kuru ||79||
prāṇāyāmaparāḥ sarve prāṇāyāmaparāyaṇāḥ |
prāṇāyāmaviśuddhā ye te yānti paramāṁ gatim ||80||
prāṇāyāmādṛte nānyattārakaṁ narakādapi |
saṁsārārṇavamagnānāṁ tārakaḥ prāṇasaṁyamaḥ ||81||
tasmāttvaṁ vidhimārgeṇa nityaṁ karma samācara |
vidhinoktena mārgeṇa prāṇasaṁyamanaṁ kuru ||82||
iti śrīyogayājñavalkye ṣaṣṭho'dhyāyaḥ ||

Therefore, you too, beautiful [Gārgī], adhere to your daily duties (in accordance with the Vedas). At all times, or during the three sandhis (morning, afternoon and evening), practice the control of prāṇa.

All those who practice prāṇāyāma regularly, with prāṇāyāma as their goal, and have been purified through prāṇāyāma, attain liberation.[66] There is no other means except prāṇāyāma to save a person from bondage.

Prāṇāyāma is the means for people who are bound in the ocean of bondage (saṁsāra) to cross over. Therefore in the prescribed manner do your daily duties (as prescribed by the Vedas) and practice prāṇāyāma in the prescribed manner.

---

[66] "tapo na paraḥ prāṇāyāmāt," that is, "there is no tapas superior to the practice of prāṇāyāma," said Manu. The same point is mentioned by Vyāsa in the Yogasūtra (II.52), while describing the benefits of the practice of prāṇāyāma. Yājñavalkya here stresses the same.

Appendix to Chapter 6

The following verses were found in other various recensions of the Yoga Yājñavalkya by Sri Divanji, the editor of the Sanskrit critical edition. These verses had no counterparts in the original manuscript which he used to compile and compare the various recensions. In some of those recensions, the following verses were placed under verse 4 of the present chapter.

Outline[67]

1-3. Meditation on Śiva

nāsāgre dṛk sadā samyak savye nyasyetaraṁ karam |
nāsāgre śaśabhṛdbimbe jyotsanājālavitānake ||1||
ambomā sahitaṁ śubhraṁ somasūryāgnilocanam |
pañcavaktraṁ mahādevaṁ candraśekharamīsvaram ||2||
nandivāhanasaṁyuktaṁ sarvadevasamanvitam |
prasannaṁ sarvavaradaṁ dhyāyetsarvāyudhaṁ śivam ||3||

Always gazing well at the tip of the nose, placing the right hand on the left, one must meditate at the tip of the nose, in the disc of the moon surrounded by its rays, on Śiva, the Divine, with eyes radiating like the sun, moon and fire, with five faces, the greatest among the deities, pure white, and bearing the moon on his head, along with Umā, the mother of all, along with his mount Nandi, surrounded by all the devas, gracious, bestowing all boons, and bearing all weapons.

4-10. Meditation on Divine represented by praṇava and gāyatrī mantra

yo vedādau svaraḥ prokto vedānte ca pratiṣṭhitaḥ |
akāramūrtireteṣāṁ raktāṅgī haṁsavāhinī ||4||
daṇḍahastā satī bālā gāyatrītyavadhāryatām |

---

[67] Yājñavalkya explains in detail how to meditate on OM using the gāyatrī mantra during sandhyāvandana, a daily ritual.

ukāramūrtireteṣāṁ kṛṣṇāṅgī vṛṣavāhanī ||5||
cakrahastā satī caiva sāvitrītyavadhāryatām |
makāramūrtireteṣāṁ śvetāṅgī tārkṣyavāhinī ||6||
śūlānandamayī vṛddhā sarasvatyavadhāryatām |
māheśvarīti sā prājñaiḥ paścimā parikīrtitā ||7||
sṛṣṭhisthityantakālādyā makāro'pyantakātmakaḥ |
akṣaratrayamevaitatkāraṇatrayamiṣyate ||8||
trayāṇāṁ kāraṇaṁ brahma sadrūpaṁ sarvakāraṇam |
ekākṣaraṁ paraṁ jyotistamāhuḥ praṇavaṁ budhāḥ ||9||
evaṁ jñātvā vidhānena praṇavena samanvitam |
prāṇāyāmaṁ tataḥ kuryādrecapūrakakumbhakaiḥ ||10||

[Meditate upon] the Divine who is represented by the praṇava at the beginning and end of the Vedas and is established [as the highest] in the vedanta.[68]

Among these seed letters (bījākṣara) constituting the praṇava (OM), the form of "A" is to be known as a young girl, of a red hue, seated on a swan, holding a stick in her hand, [embodying] the real existent truth, [called] Gāyatrī.

Among these seed letters constituting OM, the form of "U" is to be known as one with a black hue, bearing a discus (cakra) in one hand, [embodying] the real existent truth, [called] Sāvitrī.

Among the three seed letters A, U and M constituting OM, the form of "M" is to be known as an aged woman of a white hue, mounted on an eagle, bearing a spear, the personification of bliss, [called] Sarasvatī. She is praised as Māheśvarī by the wise. [Among] creation, sustenance and destruction, "M" represents destruction.

These three bījākṣaras (seed letters, A, U, and M) are considered as the three causes (creation, sustenance and destruction). The cause for the three

---

[68] Refer the Nārāyaṇavallī of the Taittirīya Upaniṣad.

is the Brahman which is the eternally existent truth, the cause for everything, self-illumined, that is spoken of as the praṇava by the realized ones.

Having known this, thus, practice prāṇāyāma with exhale, inhale and holding (rechaka, pūraka, and kumbhaka) in the orderly manner along with praṇava.

Chapter VII

OUTLINE

1: Yājñavalkya begins his discourse on pratyāhāra—the fifth limb of yoga.

2-7: Four definitions of pratyāhāra.

8-11: A list of the eighteen vital points (marmasthānas).

12-20: The distance between the vital points.

20-21: The prāṇa must be focused and held in the vital points.

22-30: Detailed description of the procedure of drawing the prāṇa from one vital point to another.

30-31: The importance of this form of pratyāhāra and its benefits.

32-37: The means to freedom by drawing and focusing the prāṇa at certain vital points.

Chapter VII

1: Yājñavalkya begins his discourse on pratyāhāra—the fifth limb of yoga.

yājñavalkya uvāca--
uktānyetāni catvāri yogāṅgāni dvijottame |
pratyāhārādi catvāri śṛṇuṣvābhyantarāṇi ca ||1||

Yājñavalkya said:

Four limbs of yoga (yama, niyama, āsana, and prāṇāyāma) have been explained, Gārgī! Listen to the [remaining] four [limbs] beginning with pratyāhāra which are internal [practices].[69]

2-7: Four definitions of pratyāhāra.

indriyāṇāṁ vicaratāṁ viṣayeṣu svabhāvataḥ |
balādāharaṇaṁ teṣāṁ pratyāhāraḥ sa ucyate ||2||
yadyatpaśyasi tatsarvaṁ paśyedātmavadātmani |
pratyāhāraḥ sa ca prokto yogavidbhirmahātmabhiḥ ||3||
karmāṇi yāni nityāni vihitāni śarīriṇām |
teṣāmātmanyanuṣṭhānaṁ manasā yadbahirvinā ||4||
pratyāhāro bhavetso'pi yogasādhanamuttamam |
pratyāhāraḥ praśasto'yaṁ sevito yogibhiḥ sadā ||5||

---

[69] The eight limbs of yoga have been classified as external (bāhya) and internal (ābhyantara) and are presented in that order here.

Yājñavalkya classifies the first four limbs as external and the latter four as internal, while the Yogasūtra classifies the first five as external and the last three as internal. The second chapter of the Yogasūtra ends with the fifth limb (pratyāhāra). The third chapter (vibhūti pāda) begins with the internal practices. Therefore, the commentator Vyāsa says, "The five external limbs have been explained. Now dhāraṇā, the internal limb, is to be spoken of.

However, the Yogasūtra clearly explains that this classification of external and internal is relative. For example, while the last three limbs are internal in relation to the first five limbs, they are external in comparison to nirbīja samādhi (Yogasūtra III.7-8).

aṣṭādaśasu yadvāyormarmasthāneṣu dhāraṇam |
sthānātsthānātsamākṛṣya pratyāhāro nigadyate ||6||
aśvinau ca tathā brūtāṁ gārgi devabhiṣagvarau |
marmasthānāni siddhyarthaṁ śarīre yogamokṣayoḥ ||7||

The senses, by nature being drawn towards [their sensory] objects, their restraint by [conscious] effort[70] is said to be pratyāhāra.

Whatever you see, look upon all of it as [being] in the self, and as the self. This is also called pratyāhāra by great souls who have realized [the essence of] yoga.

For all beings, the mental practice of the daily duties that are prescribed (by the Vedas), devoid of external actions, is also said to be pratyāhāra.

The following pratyāhāra is the greatest yogic practice and is praised and followed by yogis always. Having drawn the prāṇa from one point to another, holding it in the eighteen vital points (marmasthānas) is spoken of as pratyāhāra. The Aśvini Kumāras who are the best among the physicians of the celestials (devas) have spoken thus of the vital points in the body, for the attainment of liberation through yoga.

8-11: A list of the eighteen vital points (marmasthānas).

tāni sarvāṇi vakṣyāmi yathāvacchṛṇu suvrate |
pādāṅguṣṭhau ca gulphau ca jaṅghāmadhye tathaiva ca ||8||
cityormūlaṁ ca jānvośca madhye corudvayasya ca |
pāyumūlaṁ tataḥ paścāddehamadhyaṁ ca meḍhrakam ||9||
nābhiśca hṛdayaṁ gārgi kaṇṭhakūpastathaiva ca |
tālumūlaṁ ca nāsāyā mūlaṁ cākṣṇośca maṇḍale ||10||
bhruvormadhyaṁ lalāṭaṁ ca mūrdhā ca munisattame |
marmasthānāni caitāni mānaṁ teṣāṁ pṛthak śṛṇu ||11||

---

[70] The word used here, "balāt," should not be taken to mean forceful suppression, but intelligent effort. That is, realizing the wavering nature of the senses, they should be intelligently brought under one's control.

I shall explain all of them in an orderly manner. Listen, disciplined [Gārgī]!

The big toes, the ankles, in the mid-shanks, the root of the calves, the knees, middle of the thighs, the root of the anus, the center of the body (dehamadhya), generative organ, the navel, the heart, and neck pit, Gārgī. Then, the root of the palate, the root of the nose, circular orb of the eyes, the center of the eyebrows, the forehead, and crown of the head. [Gārgī,] best among sages!

These are the vital points. Listen to their measurement one by one.

12-20: The distance between the vital points.

pādānmānaṁ tu gulphasya sārdhāṅgulacatuṣṭayam |
gulphājjaṅghasya madhyaṁ tu vijñeyaṁ taddaśāṅgulam ||12||
jaṅghamadhyāccityormūlaṁ yattadekādaśāṅgulam |
cityormūlādvarārohe jānuḥ syādaṅgulidvayam ||13||
jānvornavāṅgulaṁ prāhurūrumadhyaṁ munīśvarāḥ |
ūrumadhyāttathā gārgi pāyumūlaṁ navāṅgulam ||14||
dehamadhyaṁ tathā pāyormūlādardhāṅguladvayam |
dehamadhyāttathā meḍhraṁ tadvatsārdhāṅguladvayam ||15||
meḍhrānnābhiśca vijñeyā gārgi sārdhadaśāṅgulam |
caturdaśāṅgulaṁ nābherhṛnmadhyaṁ ca varānane ||16||
ṣaḍaṅgulaṁ tu hṛnmadhyātkaṇṭhakūpaṁ tathaiva ca |
kaṇṭhakūpācca jihvāyā mūlaṁ syāccaturaṅgulam ||17||
nāsāmūlaṁ tu jihvāyā mūlācca caturaṅgulaṁ |
netrasthānaṁ tu tanmūlādardhāṅgulamitīṣyate ||18||
tasmādardhāṅgulaṁ viddhi bhruvorantaramātmanaḥ |
lalāṭākhyaṁ bhruvormadhyādūrdhvaṁ syādaṅguladvayam ||19||
lalāṭādvyomasaṁjñaṁ syādaṅgulitrayameva hi |

From the big toe the distance to the ankle is four and a half aṅgulas. From the ankle to mid-shank, it is known to be ten aṅgulas. From mid-shank to the root of the calf—that [distance] is eleven aṅgulas. Beautiful [Gārgī], from the root of the calf to the knee is two aṅgulas. The greatest sages say that from the knee the mid-thigh is nine aṅgulas. From the mid-thigh, the root of the anus is nine aṅgulas. The center of the body (dehamadhya) is two and a half aṅgulas from the root of the anus. Similarly, from the center of the body the generative organ is two and a half aṅgulas. The navel should be known to be ten and a half aṅgulas [from the generative organ], Gārgī! The center of the heart (hṛdaya) is fourteen aṅgulas from the navel, beautiful [Gārgī]! In the same manner the neck-pit is six aṅgulas from the center of the heart. From the neck-pit the root of the tongue will be four aṅgulas. From the root of the tongue, the root of the nose is four aṅgulas. From that root [of the nose], the place of the eye is said to be half an aṅgula. From there, know the middle of the eyebrows to be half an aṅgula. From the middle of the eyebrows, the forehead will be two aṅgulas upwards. From the forehead, the crown of the head will be three aṅgulas only.[71]

20-21: The prāṇa must be focused and held in the vital points.

sthāneṣveteṣu manasā vāyumāropya dhārayet ||20||
sthānātsthānātsamākṛṣya pratyāhāraṁ prakurvataḥ |
sarve rogā vinaśyanti yogāḥ siddhyanti tasya vai ||21||

One must focus and retain the prāṇa, using the mind, in these vital points. In one who does pratyāhāra, drawing the prāṇa from one point to another, all diseases perish. For him yoga attains fruition.

22-30: Detailed description of the procedure of drawing the prāṇa from one vital point to another.

vadanti yoginaḥ kecidyogeṣu kuśalā narāḥ |
pratyāhāraṁ varārohe śṛṇu tvaṁ tadvadāmyaham ||22||
sampūrṇakumbhavadvāyumaṅguṣṭhānmūrdhamadhyataḥ |
dhārayedanilaṁ buddhyā prāṇāyāmapracoditaḥ ||23||

---

[71] For readers' convenience, the vital points and the distance between them are summarized in a table at the end of this chapter.

vyomarandhrātsamākṛṣya lalāṭe dhārayetpunaḥ |
lalāṭādvāyumākṛṣya bhruvormadhye nirodhayet ||24||
bhruvormadhyātsamākṛṣya netramadhye nirodhayet |
netrātprāṇaṁ samākṛṣya nāsāmūle nirodhayet ||25||
nāsāmūlāttu jihvāyā mūle prāṇaṁ nirodhayet |
jihvāmūlātsamākṛṣya kaṇṭhamūle nirodhayet ||26||
kaṇṭhamūlāttu hṛnmadhye hṛdayannābhimadhyame |
nābhimadhyātpunarmeḍhre meḍhrādvahnyālaye tataḥ ||27||
dehamadhyādgude gārgi gudādevorumūlake |
ūrumūlāttayormadhye tasmājjānvornirodhayet ||28||
citimūle tatastasmājjaṅghayormadhyame tathā |
jaṅghāmadhyātsamākṛṣya vāyuṁ gulphe nirodhayet ||29||
gulphādaṅguṣṭhayorgārgi pādayostannirodhayet |

Some skilled yogis speak of [another] pratyāhāra. Listen, beautiful [Gārgī], I will tell you [about] it. During the practice of prāṇāyāma, the prāṇa must be held by the mind from the big toe to the crown of the head, like a totally filled pot. Drawing [the prāṇa] from the crown of the head, one must focus it in the forehead. Again, drawing the prāṇa from the forehead, one must focus it between the eyebrows. Drawing [the prāṇa] from the center of the eyebrows one must focus it in center of the eyes. Drawing the prāṇa from the eyes, one must focus it in the root of the nose. From the root of the nose, one must focus the prāṇa in the root of the tongue. Drawing [the prāṇa] from the root of the tongue, one must focus it in the base of the throat (neck-pit). Drawing the prāṇa from the neck-pit, one must focus it in center of the heart, from the center of heart in the center of the navel, again from the center of the navel in the generative organ and then from the generative organ in the abode of fire (dehamadhya), from the dehamadhya (center of the body), Gārgī, in the root of the anus and from the root of the anus in the [mid-] thighs, then from the mid-thigh in the center of the knees. Then, [from the knee] one must focus the prāṇa in the root of the calf, from there in the middle of the shank, and drawing [the prāṇa] from the middle of the shank in the ankle. From the ankle, Gārgī, one must focus it (the prāṇa) in the big toes of the feet.

30-31: The importance of this form of pratyāhāra and its benefits.

sthānātsthānātsamākṛṣya yastvevam dhārayet sudhīḥ ||30||
sarvapāpaviśuddhātmā jīvedācandratārakam |
etattu yogasiddhyarthamagastyenāpi kīrtitam ||31||

The wise one who, drawing the prāṇa from point to point, focuses it in the above said manner, will be freed from all bondage and will live as long as the moon and the stars exist (will attain liberation). This [pratyāhāra] is praised as the means for the fruition of yoga even by Agastya (one of the great sages). Among the pratyāhāras, this one is considered as the best by yogis.[72]

32-37: The means to freedom by drawing and focusing the prāṇa at certain vital points.

pratyāhāreṣu sarveṣu praśastamiti yogibhiḥ |
nāḍībhyāṁ vāyumāpūrya kuṇḍalyāḥ pārśvayoḥ kṣipet ||32||
dhārayedyugapatso'pi bhavarogādvimucyate |
pūrvavadvāyumāropya hṛdayavyomni dhārayaet ||33||
so'pi yāti varārohe paramātmapadaṁ naraḥ |
vyādhayaḥ kiṁ punastasya bāhyābhyantaravartinaḥ ||34||
nāsābhyāṁ vāyumāropya pūrayitvodarasthitam |
bhruvormadhyāddṛśoḥ paścātsamāropya samāhitaḥ ||35||
dhārayetkṣaṇamātraṁ vā so'pi yāti parāṁ gatim |
kiṁ punarbahunoktena nityaṁ karma samācaran ||36||
ātmanaḥ prāṇamāropya bhruvormadhye suṣumṇayā |
yāvanmano layatyasminstāvatsaṁyamanaṁ kuru ||37||

---

[72] This is called "vāyu pratyāhāra." Pratyāhāra, combined with the practice of prāṇāyāma, is explained here as involving the techniques of stepped exhalation and suspension of the breath after exhalation. Some of the other types of pratyāhāra are principally a mental practice. Thus, there are two different methods of the practice of pratyāhāra, either with or without prāṇāyāma.

iti śrīyogayajñavalkye saptmo'dhyāyaḥ ||

Inhaling the air through the nāḍīs, one must focus the prāṇa on the sides of the kunḍalinī and retain [it there]. He (who does so) is freed from bondage.

One who, as said before, draws and focuses the prāṇa in the space of the heart, he too, beautiful [Gārgī], reaches the abode of the Divine. What then are diseases, external or internal, to him?

[The one who,] inhaling the air through both nostrils, filling the belly (chest and abdomen), and then, drawing it from the center of the eyebrows to the back of the eyes, with a focused mind, retains [it there] even for a second, he too attains the highest state.

Why say more? Doing all your daily duties, focusing the prāṇa through the suṣumnā in the center of the eyebrows, control it there till the mind is totally absorbed.

Marmasthānas: Vital Points

From	To	Distance (in aṅgulas)
Big toe	Ankle	4.5
Ankle	Mid-shank	10
Mid-shank	Root of calf	11
Root of calf	Knee	2
Knee	Mid-thigh	9
Mid-thigh	Root of anus	9
Root of anus	Center of the body	2.5
Center of body	Generative organ	2.5
Generative organ	Navel	10.5
Navel	Heart	14
Heart	Neck-pit	6
Neck-pit	Root of tongue	4
Root of tongue	Root of nose	4
Root of nose	Eye	0.5
Eye	Middle of eyebrows	0.5
Middle of eyebrows	Forehead	2
Forehead	Crown of the head	3

Chapter VIII

OUTLINE

1: Yājñavalkya begins to explain the five types of dhāraṇā.

2-4: Two definitions of dhāraṇā.

5-6: The five types of dhāraṇā.

6-8: The regions of the five forms of matter in the body.

9-13: Another opinion on the region of the five forms of matter in the body. Refutation of this opinion.

14-15: The deities to be meditated upon in each of the five regions.

15-25: Procedure, duration, and results of the five dhāraṇās.

26-27: Dissolution of effects by tracing them back to their respective causes.

28-30: Another opinion that the praṇava itself can be used to bring about this involution.

30-31: Yājñavalkya instructs Gārgī to experience this involution herself using the praṇava and the practice of prāṇāyāma.

32-35: The three doṣas attain balance by the practice of prāṇāyāma itself.

36-39: All diseases, arising from the imbalance of any of the doṣas, are cured by the practice of dhāraṇā (using prāṇāyāma).

39-40: Instruction to Gārgī to practice dhāraṇā along with her daily duties.

Chapter VIII

1: Yājñavalkya begins to explain the five types of dhāraṇā.

yājñavalkya uvāca--
athedānīṁ pravakṣyāmi dhāraṇāḥ pañca tatvataḥ |
samāhitamanāstvaṁ ca śṛṇu gārgi tapodhane ||1||

Yājñavalkya said:

Now, I shall explain the essence of the five types of dhāraṇā. Gārgī, rich in austerity, you too listen with a focused mind.

2-4: Two definitions of dhāraṇā.

yamādiguṇayuktasya manasaḥ sthitirātmani |
dhāraṇetyucyate sadbhiḥ śāstratātparyavedibhiḥ ||2||
asminbrahmapure gārgi yadidaṁ hṛdayāmbujam |
tasminnevāntarākāśe yadbāahyākāśadhāraṇam ||3||
eṣā ca dhāraṇetyuktā yogaśāstraviśāradaiḥ |
tāntrikairyogaśāstrajñairvidvadbhiśca suśikṣitaiḥ ||4||

The absorption of the mind (in the self), of one endowed with qualities such as the yamas etc. [73] is said to be dhāraṇā by those who have known the essence of the scriptures.

Gārgī, in this [body which is the] abode of the Brahman, in that internal space in the heart-lotus, holding the external space is said to be dhāraṇā by the ones conversant in the yogic scriptures, by the ones who follow the tantras, the ones who have realized the essence of the yogic scriptures, and by the well-read experts.

---

[73] Only when all the preceding limbs, from yama to pratyāhāra, are practiced, will the nāḍīs be cleansed and the practitioner attains the ability to focus the prāṇa. Without this requisite preparation, both the practice and results of dhāraṇā as described in this chapter will not fructify.

5-6: The five types of dhāraṇā.

dhāraṇāḥ pañcadhā proktāstāśca sarvāḥ pṛthak śṛṇu |
bhūmirāpastathā tejo vāyurākāśameva ca ||5||
eteṣu pañcadevānāṁ dhāraṇaṁ pañcadhocyate |

Dhāraṇā is said to be of five types. Listen to all of them one by one. The dhāraṇā on the five deities (devas, representations of the Divine), [in the regions of] earth, water, fire, air, and space are said to be the five types.

6-8: The regions of the five forms of matter in the body.

pādādijānuparyantaṁ pṛthivīsthānamucyate ||6||
ājānoḥ pāyuparyantamapāṁ sthānaṁ prakīrtitam |
āpāyorhṛdayāntaṁ yadvahnisthānaṁ taducyate ||7||
āhṛnmadhyādbhruvormadhyaṁ yāvadvāyukulaṁ smṛtam |
ābhrūmadhyāttu mūrdhāntamākāśamiti cocyate ||8||

From the feet to the knees is said to be the region of earth. From the knees to the anus is spoken of as the region of water. The region from the anus to the heart, it is said to be that of fire. From the center of the heart to the center of the eyebrows is thought of as the region of air. From the center of the eyebrows to the crown of the head is said to be [the region] of space.

9-13: Another opinion on the region of the five forms of matter in the body. Refutation of this opinion.

atra kecidvadantyanye yogapaṇḍitamāninaḥ |
ājānornābhiparyantamapāṁsthānamiti dvijāḥ ||9||
nābhimadhyādgalāntaṁ yadvahnisthānaṁ taducyate |
āgalāttu lalāṭāntaṁ vāyusthānamitīritaṁ ||10||
lalāṭādrandhraparyantamākāśasthānamucyate |
ayuktametadityuktaṁ śāstratātparyavedibhiḥ ||11||
yadi syājjvalanasthānaṁ dehamadhye varānane |
ayuktā kāraṇe vahnau kāryarūpasya saṁsthitiḥ ||12||
kāryakāraṇasaṁyoge kāryahāniḥ kathaṁ bhavet |
dṛṣṭaṁ tatkāryarūpeṣu mṛdātmakaghaṭādiṣu ||13||

On this subject, some other brahmins who think themselves to be yogic scholars say that from the knees to the navel is the region of water. [The region] from the navel to the neck is said to be the region of fire. From the neck to the forehead is said to be the region of air. From the forehead to the crown of the head is said to be the region of space.

But it is said by the ones who have known the essence of the śāstras that this [opinion] is incorrect. If the region of fire is in the center of the body (dehamadhya), beautiful [Gārgī], the manifestation of the effect, in fire which is the cause, is not right. In the union of cause and effect, how can there occur a loss of the effect? This is seen in effects like pots made of mud.

14-15: The deities to be meditated upon in each of the five regions.

pṛthivyāṁ dhārayedgārgi brahmāṇaṁ parameṣṭhinam |
viṣṇumapsvanale rudramīśvaraṁ vāyumaṇḍale ||14||
sadāśivaṁ tathā vyomni dhārayetsusamāhitaḥ |

Gārgī, in [the region of] earth, one must meditate on Brahma the creator, in the region of water on Viṣṇu, in the region of fire on Rudra, in the region of air on Īśvara. In the region of space, one must meditate on Sadāśiva (another name of Śiva) with a focused mind.

15-25: Procedure, duration, and results of the five dhāraṇās.

pṛthivyāṁ vāyumāsthāya lakāreṇa samanvitam ||15||
dhyāyaṁścaturbhujākāraṁ brahmāṇaṁ sṛṣṭikāraṇam |
dhārayetpañca ghaṭikāḥ pṛthivījayamāpnuyāt ||16||
vāruṇe vāyumāropya vakāreṇa samanvitam |
smarannārāyaṇaṁ saumyaṁ caturbāhuṁ kirīṭinam ||17||
śuddhasphatikasaṅkāśaṁ pītavāsasamacyutam |
dhārayetpañca ghaṭikāḥ sarvarogaiḥ pramucyate ||18||
vahnau cānilamāropya rephākṣarasamanvitam |
tryakṣaṁ varapradaṁ rudraṁ taruṇādityasannibham ||19||
bhasmodhdūlitasarvāṅgaṁ suprasannamanusmaran |

dhārayetpañca ghaṭikāḥ vahnināsau na dahyate ||20||
māruta mārutasthāne yakāreṇa samanvitam |
dhārayetpañca ghaṭikāḥ vāyuvadvyomago bhavet ||21||
ākāśe vāyumāropya hakāropari śaṅkaram |
bindurūpaṁ mahādevaṁ vyomākāraṁ sadāśivam ||22||
śuddhasphaṭikasaṅkāśaṁ bālendughṛtamaulinam |
pañcavaktrayutaṁ saumyaṁ daśabāhuṁ trilocanam ||23||
sarvāyudhodyatakaraṁ sarvābharaṇabhūṣitam |
umārdhadehaṁ varadaṁ sarvakāraṇakāraṇam ||24||
manasā cintayanstu muhūrtamapi dhārayet |
sa eva mukta ityuktastāntrikeṣu suśikṣitaiḥ ||25||

The one who focuses the prāṇa in [the region of] earth, with the [seed letter] "lam," meditating upon the creator Brahma, portrayed with four hands, and retains [the prāṇa] for two hours (five ghatikās) attains mastery over earth.

The one who focuses the prāṇa in the region of water, with the [seed letter] "vam," meditating on changeless Nārāyaṇa, with four hands, [bearing] a crown, pleasing [in appearance], with a hue like that of a pure crystal, wearing a yellow garment, and retains it [the prāṇa] for two hours becomes free from all diseases.

The one who focuses the prāṇa in the region of fire, with the [seed letter] "ram," meditating upon the gracious Rudra who grants boons, with three eyes, and a hue like the rising sun, [his] entire body smeared with holy ash, and retains it [the prāṇa] for two hours is not burnt by fire.

The one who focuses the prāṇa in the region of air, with the [seed letter] "yam," meditating on Ardhanārīśvara,[74] adorned with all the various ornaments, bearing all weapons in his hands, the primeval cause for everything, who grants boons, and retains [the prāṇa] for two hours, can

[74] Ardhanārīśvara is a conjoint figure of Śiva and Pārvatī, with the male form on the right side and female form on the left.

move in space, like air [moves in space].

The one who focuses the prāṇa in the region of space, with the [seed letter] "ham," meditating, using the mind, on the auspicious Sadāśiva, in the form of a bindu, the greatest of the deities, represented by space, with a hue like a pure crystal, bearing the crescent moon on his head, with ten arms, five heads, and three eyes, pleasing [in appearance], and retains [the prāṇa] for 90 minutes (one muhūrta)—such a person alone is said to have attained freedom by those well versed in the tantras.

26-27: Dissolution of effects by tracing them back to their respective causes.

etaduktaṁ bhavatyatra gārgi brahmavidāṁ vare |
brahmādikāryarūpāṇi sve sve saṁhṛtya kāraṇe ||26||
tasminsadāśive prāṇaṁ cittaṁ cānīya kāraṇe |
yuktacittastadātmānaṁ yojayetparameśvare ||27||

Gārgī! Best among those who have realized the Brahman! This is [the essence of] what is said here. Dissolving the manifestations, like the forms such as Brahmā etc. in their respective causes, absorbing the prāṇa and the mind in that Sadāśiva who is the cause [for everything], with a concentrated mind, one must unite the self with the Divine.

28-30: Another opinion that the praṇava itself can be used to bring about this involution.

asminnarthe vadantyanye yogino brahmavidvarāḥ |
praṇavenaiva kāryāṇi sve sve saṁhṛtya kāraṇe ||28||
praṇavasya tu nādānte paramāndavigraham |
ṛtaṁ satyaṁ paraṁ brahma puruṣaṁ kṛṣṇapiṅgalam ||29||
cetasā saṁprapaśyanti santaḥ saṁsārabheṣajam |

In this matter, other yogis who are the greatest among those who have realized the Brahman, say, "Dissolving the manifestations in their respective causes, using the praṇava with a clear mind, at the end of the sound of the praṇava, the wise perceive the Self, the eternal, unchanging

Brahman, the personification of bliss and the cure for bondage,[75] in a hue of red and black."

30-31: Yājñavalkya instructs Gārgī to experience this involution herself using the praṇava and the practice of prāṇāyāma.

tvaṁ tasmāt praṇavenaiva prāṇāyāmaistribhistribhiḥ ||30||
brahmādi kāryarūpāṇi sve sve saṁhṛtya kāraṇe |
viśuddha cetasā paśya nādānte parameśvaram ||31||

Therefore [Gārgī], you too perceive the Divine, by practising prāṇāyāma in threes and threes,[76] dissolving the manifestations like the forms such as Brahma etc., in their respective causes using the praṇava, with a clear mind, at the end of the sound [of the praṇava].

32-35: The three doṣas attain balance by the practice of prāṇāyāma itself.

asminnarthe vadantyanye yogino brahmavidvarāḥ |
bhiṣagvarā varārohe yogeṣu pariniṣṭhitāḥ ||32||
śarīraṁ tāvadevaṁ tu pañcabhūtātmakaṁ khalu |
tadetattu varārohe vātapittakaphātmakam ||33||
vātātmakānāṁ sarveṣāṁ yogeṣvabhiratātmanām |
prāṇasaṁyamanenaiva śoṣaṁ yāti kalevaram ||34||
pittātmakānāṁ tvacirānna śuṣyati kalevaram |
kaphātmakānāṁ kāyaśca sampūrṇastvacirādbhavet ||35||

Beautiful [Gārgī], in this matter, other yogis, who are the greatest among those who have realized the Brahman, the greatest physicians, and experts on yoga say [thus].

The body is made of the five forms of matter is it not, beautiful [Gārgī]?

---

[75] Up to this point, Yājñavalkya has described dhāraṇā on deities with form and attributes. Now, dhāraṇā using OM is described.

[76] This refers to three rounds of 6 breaths each, practiced three times a day (in the morning, afternoon and evening).

That body also has the three doṣas (vāta, pitta, kapha).

In those absorbed in [the practice of] yoga in whom vāta is dominant, the body dries up by the practice of prāṇāyāma itself. In those in whom pitta is dominant, the body does not dry up easily and the body of those in whom kapha is dominant becomes well-nourished quickly.

36-39: All diseases, arising from the imbalance of any of the doṣas, are cured by the practice of dhāraṇā (using prāṇāyāma).

dhāraṇaṁ kurvatastvagnau sarve naśyanti vātajāḥ |
pārthivāṁśe jalāṁśe ca dhāraṇaṁ kurvataḥ sadā ||36||
naśyanti śleṣmajā rogā vātajāścācirāttathā |
vyomāṁśe mārutāṁśe ca dhāraṇaṁ kurvataḥ sadā ||37||
tridoṣajanitā rogā vinaśyanti na saṁśayaḥ |
asminnarthe tathābrūtāmaśvinau ca bhiṣagvarāḥ ||38||
prāṇasaṁyamanenaiva tridoṣaśamanaṁ nṛṇām |

In one who does dhāraṇā on fire, all [diseases] caused by vāta perish.

In one who always does dhāraṇā on the aspects of earth and water, diseases arising from kapha and vāta perish soon.[77]

In one who always does dhāraṇā on the aspects of space and air, diseases arising from any of the three doṣas are destroyed.

In this matter, the Aśvini Kumāras who are the best among physicians say thus.[78] Only through the control of prāṇa is there a balancing of the three doṣas in [all] human beings.

---

[77] Another recension reads here: "those caused by vāta and pitta perish."

[78] The imbalance of the three doṣas can be corrected, and diseases can be cured using the practice of dhāraṇā, by focusing the mind on the regions of the five elements in the body, along with the practice of prāṇāyāma.

39-40: Instruction to Gārgī to practice dhāraṇā along with her daily duties.

tasmāttvaṁ ca varārohe nityaṁ karma samācara ||39||
yamādibhiśca samyuktā vidhivaddhāraṇaṁ kuru ||40||
iti śrīyogayājñavalkye aṣṭamo'dhyāyaḥ ||

Therefore you too, beautiful [Gārgī], do your daily duties (in accordance with the Vedas). Do dhāraṇā in a proper manner, along with the yamas etc. (along with all the preceeding limbs of yoga).

Division of Body into Various Regions Representing Forms of Matter and the Seed Letter Mantras

Yoga Yājñavalkya, Chapter VIII (6-8)

REGION	FORM OF MATTER	MANTRA
Feet to knees	Earth	Lam
Knees to generative organ	Water	Vam
Generative organ to heart	Fire	Ram
Heart to center of eyebrows	Air	Yam
Center of eyebrows to crown of the head	Space	Ham

Mantra Mahodadhi I.14-18 (From the text, "Ocean of Mantras")

REGION	FORM OF MATTER	MANTRA
Feet to knees	Earth	Lam
Knees to navel	Water	Vam
Navel to heart	Fire	Ram
Heart to center of eyebrows	Air	Yam
Center of eyebrows to crown of the head	Space	Ham

Chapter IX

OUTLINE

1: Yājñavalkya begins his discourse on dhyāna.

2: Definition of dhyāna. The two types of dhyāna: saguṇa (with attributes) and nirguṇa (without attributes).

3: The number of types in each form of dhyāna.

4: The prerequisites for dhyāna.

5-9: Description of dhyāna without attributes (nirguṇa).

10-11: Another form of dhyāna without attributes (nirguṇa dhyāna).

12-18: Dhyāna with attributes (saguṇa) on the Divine in the form of Nārāyaṇa.

19-24: Dhyāna with attributes on the Divine (saguṇa) in the form of Vaiśvānara Agni in one's own body.

25-30: Dhyāna with attributes (saguṇa) on the Divine in the disc of the sun.

31-32: Dhyāna on one's self.

32-34: Dhyāna on the Divine in the space between the eyebrows.

35-39: Another form of saguṇa dhyāna on one's own self in the heart-lotus.

40-41: Benefits of dhyāna.

42-44: Instruction to Gārgī to practice dhyāna, along with her daily duties.

Chapter IX

1: Yājñavalkya begins his discourse on dhyāna.

yājñavalkya uvāca--
atha dhyānaṁ pravakṣyāmi śṛṇu gārgi varānane |
dhyānameva hi jantūnāṁ kāraṇaṁ bandhamokṣayoḥ ||1||

Now, I will explain dhyāna. Beautiful Gārgī, listen to me. Dhyāna alone is the cause for bondage or freedom of all beings.[79]

2: Definition of dhyāna. The two types of dhyāna: saguṇa (with attributes) and nirguṇa (without attributes).

dhyānamātmasvarūpasya vedanaṁ manasā khalu |
saguṇaṁ nirguṇaṁ tacca saguṇaṁ bahuśaḥ smṛtam ||2||

Dhyāna is to know (realize) the self through the mind. Dhyāna may be devoid of attributes (nirguṇa) or with attributes (saguṇa). Dhyāna with attributes (saguṇa) is further thought to be of several types.

3: The number of types in each form of dhyāna.

pañcottamāni teṣvāhurvaidikāni dvijottamāḥ |
trīṇi mukhyatamānyeṣāmekameva hi nirguṇaṁ ||3||

Among these [types of saguṇa dhyāna], the best among brahmins say that five [types] which are in accordance with the Vedas, are important, and among these [five], three are most important, while dhyāna devoid of attributes (nirguṇa) is only one.

4: The prerequisites for dhyāna.

marmasthānāni nāḍīnāṁ saṁsthānaṁ ca pṛthakpṛthak |
vāyūnāṁ sthānakarmāṇi jñātvā kurvātmavedanaṁ ||4||

After knowing properly the marmasthānas, the position of the nāḍīs, and

---

[79] It is important to note that meditation can lead to bondage.

the position and function of the vāyus,[80] undertake the realization of the self.

5-9: Description of dhyāna without attributes (nirguṇa).

ekaṁ jyotirmayaṁ śuddhaṁ sarvagam vyomavaddṛḍham |
avyaktamacalaṁ nityamādimadhyāntavarjitam ||5||
sthūlam sūkṣmamanākāramasaṁspṛśyamacākṣuṣam |
na rasaṁ na ca gandhākhyamaprameyamanaupamam ||6||
ānandamajaraṁ nityaṁ sadasatsarvakāraṇam |
sarvādhāraṁ jagadrūpamamūrtamajamavyayam ||7||
adṛśyaṁ dṛśyamantaḥsthaṁ bahiḥsthaṁ sarvatomukham |
sarvadṛksarvataḥpādaṁ sarvaspṛk sarvataḥśiraḥ ||8||
brahma brahmamayo'haṁ syāmiti yadvedanaṁ bhavet |
tadetannirguṇaṁ dhyānamiti brahmavido viduḥ ||9||

I am the Brahman, effulgent, pure, all pervading like space, unmanifest, steady and eternal, with no beginning, middle, or end, gross and subtle, formless, beyond touch or sight through the eyes, beyond taste and smell, beyond perception [through the senses], unequalled, blissful, imperishable, eternal, the cause for all, both manifest and unmanifest, the basis for everything, pervading the entire world, without beginning, devoid of change, seen and unseen, present inside and outside, existing in all forms, omnipresent.[81] Such realization is known to be dhyāna without attributes (nirguṇa) by those who have realized the Brahman.

10-11: Another form of dhyāna without attributes (nirguṇa dhyāna).

athavā paramātmānaṁ paramānandavigraham |
gurūpadeśādvijñāya puruṣaṁ kṛṣṇapiṅgalam ||10||

---

[80] Yājñavalkya again emphasizes that, if dhyāna is to succeed, one must be well versed in all the practices discussed in the previous chapters.

[81] The same concept is expressed in the Bhagavad Gīta in many verses, for example in XII.13-14.

brahma brahmapure cāsmindaharāmbujamadhyame |
abhyāsātsamprapaśyanti santaḥ saṁsārabheṣajam ||11||

Otherwise, through initiation from a guru, having understood the Divine, the personification of bliss, in a red and black form, in this residence of the Brahman (in this body), the wise clearly experience the Brahman, the cure for bondage, in the center of the heart-lotus through continuous practice.

12-18: Dhyāna with attributes (saguṇa) on the Divine in the form of Nārāyaṇa.

hṛtpadme'ṣṭadalopete kandamadhyātsamutthite |
dvādaśāṅgulanāle'smiṁścaturaṅgulamunmukhe ||12||
prāṇāyāmairvikāsite kesarānvitakarṇike |
vāsudevaṁ jagannāthaṁ nārāyaṇamajaṁ harim ||13||
caturbhujamudārāṅgaṁ śaṅkhacakragadādharam |
kirīṭakeyūradharaṁ padmapatranibhekṣaṇam ||14||
śrīvatsavakṣasaṁ viṣṇuṁ pūrṇacandranibhānanam |
padmodaradalābhoṣṭhaṁ suprasannaṁ śucismitam ||15||
śuddhasphaṭikasaṅkāśaṁ pītavāsasamacyutam |
padmacchavipadadvandvaṁ paramātmānamavyayam ||16||
prabhābhirbhāsayadrūpaṁ paritaḥ puruṣottamam |
manasālokya deveśaṁ sarvabhūtahṛdi sthitam ||17||
so'hamātmeti vijñānaṁ saguṇaṁ dhyānamucyate |

In the heart-lotus with eight petals, rising from the center of the kandasthāna with a stalk of twelve aṅgulas and facing four more aṅgulas upwards, with filaments and pericarp, which has bloomed due to [the practice of] prāṇāyāma,[82] [who is known as] Nārāyaṇa, Vāsudeva, Hari, Viṣṇu, Acyuta (epithets), beyond birth, the lord of the universe, with four arms, of pleasing form, bearing a conch, discus and mace, adorned with armlets and a crown, with eyes like the petals of a lotus, bearing the mole

---

[82] Note the continued importance placed upon the practice of prāṇāyāma.

called Śrīvatsa[83] on his chest, his face as beautiful as the full moon, lips like the petals of a lotus, gracious, with a charming smile, his hue like that of a pure crystal, clothed in yellow, with feet like lotus, unchanging, Divine, illuminating all by his effulgence, the Supreme Being and the lord of the celestials, present in the heart of all beings—seeing him with the mind, with the realization that "He is I (the self)" is said to be dhyāna with attributes (saguṇa).

19-24: Dhyāna with attributes on the Divine (saguṇa) in the form of Vaiśvānara Agni in one's own body.

hṛtsaroruhamadhye'sminprakṛtyātmakakarṇike ||18||
aṣṭaiśvaryadalopete vidyākesarasaṁyute |
jñānanāle bṛhatkande prāṇāyāmaprabodhite ||19||
viśvārciṣaṁ mahāvahniṁ jvalantaṁ viśvatomukham |
vaiśvānaraṁ jagadyoniṁ śikhātanvinamīśvaram ||20||
tāpayantaṁ svakaṁ dehamāpādatalamastakam |
nirvātadīpavattasmindīpitaṁ havyavāhanam ||21||
dṛṣṭvā tasya śikhāmadhye paramātmānamakṣaram |
nīlatoyadamadhyasthavidyullekheva bhāsvaram ||22||
nīvāraśūkavadrūpaṁ pītābhaṁ sarvakāraṇam |
jñātvā vaiśvānaraṁ devaṁ so'hamātmeti yā matiḥ ||23||
saguṇeṣūttamaṁ hyetaddhyānaṁ yogavido viduḥ |
vaiśvānaratvaṁ samprāpya muktiṁ tenaiva gacchati ||24||

In the center of the heart-lotus, with the seen (prakṛti) as its pericarp, the eight siddhis as its petals, and realization (jñāna) as its filament, with the stalk of realization, and the Divine (Paramatma) as its base of origin, which has bloomed due to [the practice of] Prāṇāyāma.

By whose effulgence, the entire world is luminescent, the great fire of knowledge which annihilates the ego, the one who is present everywhere,

---

[83] This represents the Goddess Lakṣmī.

the cause of the world, known as Vaiśvānara, in the form of a flame, luminescent from head to toe, whose flame is as steady as that of a lamp shining in a place without wind, who shines like fire, after seeing and knowing in the middle of the fine flame, the Divine, imperishable, resplendent like a bolt of lightning in the middle of a blue sea, yellow in hue and in form as slender as the tip of a grain of rice, who is the source of everything, the lord, also known as Vaiśvānara—having known thus, the realization that "He is I (the self)" is the best among all qualities and this is dhyāna according to those well-versed in yoga.

By this dhyāna itself, one attains unity with the Divine[84] (in the form of Vaiśvānara) and becomes liberated.[85]

25-30: Dhyāna with attributes (saguṇa) on the Divine in the disc of the sun.

athavā maṇḍale paśyedādityasya mahādyuteḥ |
ātmānaṁ sarvajagataḥ puruṣaṁ hema rūpiṇam ||25||
hiraṇyaśmaśrukeśaṁ ca hiraṇyamayanakhaṁ harim |
kanakāmbujavadvaktraṁ sṛṣṭisthityantakāraṇam ||26||
padmāsanasthitaṁ saumyaṁ prabuddhābjanibhānanam |
padmodaradalābhākṣaṁ sarvalokābhayapradam ||27||
jānantaṁ sarvadā sarvamunnayantaṁ ca dhārmikān |
bhāsayantaṁ jagatsarvaṁ dṛṣṭvā lokaikasākṣiṇam ||28||
so'hamasmīti yā buddhiḥ sa ca dhyāneṣu śasyate |
eṣa eva tu mokṣasya mahāmārgastapodhane ||29||
dhyānenānena saureṇa muktiṁ yāsyanti sūrayaḥ |
bhruvormadhye'ntarātmānaṁ bhārūpaṁ sarvakāraṇam ||30||

Otherwise, one must see in the disc of the luminous sun, Hari (an epithet of

---

[84] In the Bhagavad Gīta, Krishna refers to being present as the Divine in one and all as the vaiśvānara agni (XVI.14).

[85] The same concept has been expressed in the Nārāyaṇavallī of the Taittirīya Upaniṣad.

Viṣṇu) who is the self (ātma) of [all beings in] the whole world, golden in form, with golden hair, moustache and nails, who removes all sins, with a face like a golden lotus, the basis for creation, sustenance and destruction, seated in padmāsana, peaceful, whose face has the beauty of a fully-bloomed lotus, with eyes like the leaves of a lotus, the protector of all the worlds, all-knowing at all times, who uplifts those who do their dharma, illuminating the entire world, a witness to all that goes on in the world.

After seeing him, the realization that "He is I (the self)" is most praiseworthy among the various forms of dhyāna. This is the best way to freedom, [Gārgī], rich in austerity!

31-32: Dhyāna on one's self.

sthāṇuvanmūrdhaparyantaṁ madhyadehātmasamutthitam |
jagatkāraṇamavyaktaṁ jvalantamamitaujasam ||31||
manasālokya so'haṁ syāmityetaddhyānamuttamam |
Wise men attain freedom by this Dhyāna on the Divine in the sun. Seeing with the mind in the middle of the eyebrows, the Divine, that is effulgent, the source of everything, arising from the center of the body and extending up to the head like a pillar, the basis of the world, causeless, and of immeasurable splendour, the meditation that "He is I (the self)" is the best form of dhyāna.

32-34: Dhyāna on the Divine in the space between the eyebrows.

athavā baddhaparyaṅke śitilīkṛtavigrahe ||32||
śiva eva svayaṁ bhūtvā nāsāgrāropitekṣaṇaḥ |
nirvikāraṁ paraṁ śāntaṁ paramātmānamīśvaraṁ ||33||
bhārūpamamṛtam dhyāyedbhruvormadhye varānane |
so'hameveti yā buddhiḥ sā ca dhyāneṣu śasyate ||34||

Otherwise, seated firmly in padmāsana, with the body relaxed, with the intention of uniting with Śiva (one form of the Divine), gazing of the tip of the nose, one must meditate upon the Divine in the center of the eyebrows, who is beyond any change, peaceful, all-powerful, effulgent and imperishable.

The realization that "He is I (the self)" is the most praiseworthy among the various forms of Dhyāna, beautiful [Gārgī]!

35-39: Another form of saguna dhyāna on one's own self in the heart-lotus.

athavāṣṭadalopete karṇikākesarānvite |
unnidrahṛdayāmbhoje somamaṇḍalamadhyame ||35||
svātmānamarbhakākaraṁ bhoktṛrūpiṇamavyayam |
sudhārasaṁ vimuñcadbhiḥ śaśiraśmibhirāvṛtam ||36||
ṣoḍaśacchadasaṁyuktaśiraḥpadmādadhomukhāt |
nirgatāmṛtadhārābhiḥ sahasrābhiḥ samantataḥ ||37||
plāvitaṁ puruṣaṁ tatra cintayitvā samāhitaḥ |
tenāmṛtarasenaiva sāṅgopāṅgakalevare ||38||
ahameva paraṁ brahma paramātmāhamavyayaḥ |
evaṁ yadvedanaṁ tacca saguṇaṁ dhyānamucyate ||39||

Otherwise, in the fully-bloomed heart-lotus, with eight petals, pericarp, and filament, [visualizing it to be] the center of the disc of the moon, thinking of one's own self, unchanging, in a minute form, surrounded by the rays of the moon emanating nectar, surrounded on all sides by the thousands of rays of nectar emanating from his head which is in the form of an inverted lotus with sixteen petals, in this body with all its limbs, with a totally focused mind, the realization that "I am the Divine (Brahman). I am eternal and unchanging." is said to be saguṇa dhyāna.

40-41: Benefits of dhyāna.

evaṁ dhyānāmṛtam kurvan ṣanmāsānmṛtyujidbhavet |
vatsarānmukta eva syājjīvanneva na saṁśayaḥ ||40||
jīvanmuktasya na kvāpi duḥkhāvāptiḥ kathañcana |
kiṁ punarnityamuktasya muktireva hi durlabhā ||41||

One who does dhyāna thus (in any one of the above said manners) for six months, vanquishes death. In one year, he undoubtedly becomes liberated, even when alive. One who has attained freedom is never afflicted by sorrow anywhere. Then why speak of the yogi who is eternally free?

42-44: Instruction to Gārgī to practice dhyāna, along with her daily duties.

tasmāttvam ca varārohe phalam tyaktvaiva nityaśaḥ |
vidhivatkarma kurvāṇā dhyānameva sadā kuru ||42||
anyānapi bahūnyāhurdhyānāni munisattamāḥ |
mukhyānyuktāni caitebhyo jaghanyānītarāṇi tu ||43||
saguṇaṁ guṇahīnaṁ vā vijñāyātmānamātmani |
santaḥ samādhiṁ kurvanti tvamapyevaṁ sadā kuru ||44||
iti śrīyogayājñavalkye navamo'dhyāyaḥ ||

Therefore, you too, beautiful Gārgī, doing all your prescribed actions, having relinquished the desire for the results, do dhyāna at all times. Great sages have spoken of many other types of dhyāna. But the most important ones have been described above and the others are not as important.

Whether with attributes (saguṇa) or without attributes (nirguṇa), great seers realize the self within themselves leading to samādhi. You too always practice thus.

Chapter X

OUTLINE

1: Yājñavalkya begins to speak on samādhi, which destroys all bondage.

2: Samādhi is defined as the state of union of the self and the Divine.

3-5: One attains samādhi (becomes one) with the object on which one does dhyāna. Dhyāna culminates in samādhi. Surrender also leads to samādhi.

6-9: The prerequisites for attaining samādhi.

9-18: The process by which a yogi attains samādhi and leaves his body.

18-19: One should leave one's body thinking of that upon which one has focused during the practice of yoga.

19-20: One becomes that which one thinks of during the time of death.

20-21: Instructions to Gārgī on the manner of leaving the body.

21-22: Freedom is assured for one who follows the actions laid down in the Vedas without desire.

22-24: Yājñavalkya concludes his explanation of the path of yoga.

Chapter X

1: Yājñavalkya begins to speak on samādhi, which destroys all bondage.

yājñavalkya uvāca--
samādhimadhunā vakṣye bhavapāśavināśanam |
bhavapāśanibaddhasya yathāvacchrotumarhasi ||1||

Yājñavalkya said, "I will now speak about samādhi which destroys all the ties of worldly bondage of one who is bound by worldly ties. Listen in the proper manner."

2: Samādhi is defined as the state of union of the self and the Divine.

samādhiḥ samatāvasthā jīvātmaparamātmanoḥ |
brahmaṇyeva sthitiryāa sā samādhiḥ pratyagātmanaḥ ||2||

The state of unity of the self and the Divine is samādhi. The state [of absorption] of the self in the Brahman is samādhi.

3-5: One attains samādhi (becomes one) with the object on which one does dhyāna. Dhyāna culminates in samādhi. Surrender also leads to samādhi.

dhyāyedyathā yathātmānaṁ tatsamādhistathā tathā |
dhyātvaivātmani saṁsthāpyo nānyathātmā yathā bhavet ||3||
evameva tu sarvatra yatprapannastu yo naraḥ |
tadātmā so'pi tatraiva samādhiṁ samavāpnuyāt ||4||
sāritpatau niviṣṭāmbu yathābhinnatayānviyāt |
tathātmābhinna evātra samādhiṁ samavāpnuyāt ||5||

In whichever way one does dhyāna on whatever object, that culminates in samādhi. Therefore, one must meditate on the self, so that one realizes the self.

Similarly, the person who, in all places, has surrendered to a certain object and is absorbed in that object, he too attains a state of samādhi.

Just as the water which enters the sea (from the rivers) attains oneness [with the sea], similarly, one attains oneness with the self and reaches [the state of] samādhi.

6-9: The prerequisites for attaining samādhi.

etaduktaṁ bhavatyatra gārgi brahmavidāṁ vare |
karmaiva vidhivatkurvankāmasaṅkalpavarjitam ||6||
vedānteṣvatha śāstreṣu suśikṣitamanāḥ sadā |
guruṇā tūpadiṣṭārthaṁ yuktyupetaṁ varānane ||7||
vidvadbhirdharmaśāstrajñairvicārya ca punaḥ punaḥ |
tasminsuniścitārtheṣu suśikṣitamanāḥ sadā ||8||

Beautiful Gārgī! Greatest among those who have realized the Brahman! This is [the essence] said here. Doing all the actions laid down in the Vedas, without the motivation of desire, with a mind well trained in all the scriptures including vedānta, with intellegent reflection on that into which one has been initiated by the guru, having deeply reflected repeatedly with scholars and those proficient in the Vedic scriptures which lay down the proper way of life, and having imbibed deeply in one's mind the essence of these, one must always strive for the union of the self and the Divine.

9-18: The process by which a yogi attains samādhi and leaves his body.

yogamevābhyasennityaṁ jīvātmaparamātmanoḥ
|tatastvābhyantaraiścihnairbāhyairvā kālasūcakaiḥ ||9||
viniścityātmanaḥ kālamanyairvā paramārthavit |
nirbhayaḥ suprasannātmā martyastu vijitendriyaḥ ||10||
svakarmanirataḥ śāntaḥ sarvabhūtahite rataḥ |
pradāya vidyāṁ putrasya mantraṁ ca vidhipūrvakam ||11||
saṁskāramātmanaḥ sarvamupadiśya tadānaghe |
puṇyakṣetre śucau deśe vidvadbhiśca samāvṛte ||12||
bhūmau kuśānsamāstīrya kṛṣṇājinamathāpi vā |
tasminsubaddhaparyaṅko mantrairbaddhakalevaraḥ ||13||
āsane nānyadhīrāste prāṅmukho vāpyudaṅmukhaḥ |
navadvārāṇi saṁyamya gārgyasminbrahmaṇaḥ pure ||14||

unnidrahṛdayāmbhoje prāṇāyāmaiḥ prabodhite |
vyomni tasminprabhārūpe svarūpe sarvakāraṇe ||15||
manovṛttiṁ susaṁyamya paramātmani paṇḍitaḥ |
mūrdhnyādhāyātmanaḥ prāṇaṁ bhruvormadhye'thavānaghe ||16||
kāraṇe paramānande āsthito yogadhāraṇām |
omityekākṣaraṁ buddhyā vyāharansusamāhitaḥ ||17||
śarīraṁ saṁtyajedvidvānātmaivābhūnnarottamaḥ |

Then, by signs internal, external or otherwise, signifying the approach of death, having clearly determined [the time of] death, the person, who has realized the highest truth, being free from fear, with a pleasant disposition, having conquered all the senses, and is devoted to the performance of his duties, totally peaceful and interested in the welfare of all beings, after imparting his knowledge and mantra to his son (or student) in the prescribed manner, and after initiating him into the means for purification of oneself, then, pure [Gārgī], in an auspicious place, in a clean environment, surrounded by learned men, spreading kuśa grass (a special variety of grass) or deerskin on the ground, sitting firmly in padmāsana, having controlled his body by the use of mantras, with a mind that is not distracted, facing east or north, having closed the nine openings [of the body] (exits of the prāṇa), Gārgī, in this [body which is the] abode of the Brahman, in the fully-bloomed heart-lotus, awakened by prāṇāyāma, directing the activities of the mind on the luminous form of the Divine who is the cause for everything, who is one's self, in that space [of the heart-lotus], the learned one, drawing his prāṇa to the crown of the head, or in between his eyebrows, pure [Gārgī], with a mind focused through the practice of yoga, in that which is the cause [for everything], which is [the personification of] bliss, mentally saying the single syllable "OM," the learned person should give up his body. [Such a person,] the most illustrious among men, becomes one with the self.

18-19: One should leave one's body thinking of that upon which one has focused during the practice of yoga.

yasminsamabhyasedvidvānyogenaivātmadarśanaṁ ||18||
tadeva samsmaranvidvāṁstyajedante kalevaram |

He should give up the body, thinking of that upon which he has focused during the practice of yoga, and attained the knowledge of the self.

19-20: One becomes that which one thinks of during the time of death.

yaṁ yaṁ samyaksmaranbhāvaṁ tyajatyante kalevaram ||19||
tam tamevaityasau bhāvamiti yogavido viduḥ |

Whatever a person thinks of at the time of leaving his body (death), he becomes that. Thus say the ones who have known the essence of yoga.[86]

20-21: Instructions to Gārgī on the manner of leaving the body.

tvaṁ caivaṁ yogamāsthāya dhyāyansvātmānamātmani ||20||
svadharmaniratā śāntā tyajānte dehamātmanaḥ |

You too, firmly established in the practice of yoga, meditating upon the self in you, performing all your duties in accordance with the Vedas, remaining totally peaceful, leave your body finally.

21-22: Freedom is assured for one who follows the actions laid down in the Vedas without desire.

jñānenaiva sahaitena nityakarmāṇi kurvataḥ ||21||
nivṛttaphalasaṅgasya muktirgārgi kare sthitā |

Gārgī! Freedom is in the hands of the one who continues to perform all his daily duties, along with such realization, and who has relinquished the desire for the fruits [of the actions].

---

[86] The same concept is explained in the Bhagavad Gita (VIII.6) in almost the same words.

22-24: Yājñavalkya concludes his explanation of the path of yoga.

yaduktaṁ brahmaṇā pūrvaṁ karmayogasamuccayam ||22||
tadetatkīrtitam sarvaṁ sāṅgopāṅgaṁ vidhānataḥ |
tvaṁ caiva yogamabhyasya yamādyaṣṭāṅgasamyutam ||23||
nirvāṇaṁ padamāsādya prapañcaṁ saṁparityaja ||24||
iti śrīyogayājñavalkye daśamo'dhyāyaḥ ||

The link between action (karma) and realization (yoga or jñāna) which was mentioned by Brahma earlier,[87] has been expounded in the proper manner, with all its limbs and auxiliary limbs. You too, thus practising yoga, with the eight limbs starting from yama, attain the state of freedom (nirvāṇa), and completely give up the world.

[87] Yājñavalkya here refers to his earlier conversation with Brahma (see I.27).

Chapter XI

OUTLINE

1-2: Gārgī requests Yājñavalkya to explain the purification for not having performed the Vedic duties (prāyaścitta) when in a state of yoga (samādhi).

3-6: Yājñavalkya's reply that when one is in yoga (samādhi), no purification is needed later for not doing Vedic or other duties (prāyaścitta).

7-10: When not in a state of yoga (samādhi), even a realized person must do all the Vedic duties.

10-12: Instruction to Gārgī to attain freedom through the practice of yoga. Yājñavalkya's request to all the sages to return to their respective hermitages.

13-16: The sages return to their respective hermitages, after duly saluting Yājñavalkya.

16-19: Gārgī's request to Yājñavalkya to explain the whole of yoga with all its eight limbs concisely.

20-22: Yājñavalkya's consent to explain the path of yoga concisely.

Chapter XI

1-2: Gārgī requests Yājñavalkya to explain the purification for not having performed the Vedic duties (prāyaścitta) when in a state of yoga (samādhi).

ityevamuktā muninā yājñavalkyena dhīmatā |
ṛṣimadhye varārohā vākyametadabhāṣata ||1||
gārgyuvāca--
yogayukto naraḥ svāminsandhyayorvāthavā sadā |
vaidhaṁ karma kathaṁ kuryānniṣkṛtiḥ kā tvakurvataḥ ||2||

Told thus by the wise sage Yājñavalkya, the beautiful [Gārgī], spoke as follows in the midst of the sages.

Gārgī said, "Master, how will a person who is involved in the practice of yoga do the actions prescribed by the Vedas during the sandhis or always? What is the prāyaścitta (an action of purification for not having performed the prescribed Vedic duties) for one who does not do them?"

3-6: Yājñavalkya's reply that when one is in yoga (samādhi), no purification is needed later for not doing Vedic or other duties (prāyaścitta).

ityukto brahmavādinyā brahmavidbrāhmaṇastadā |
tāṁ samālokya bhagavānidamāha narottamaḥ ||3||
yājñavalkya uvāca--
yogayuktamanuṣyasya sandhyayorvāthavā niśi |
yatkartavyaṁ varārohe yogena khalu tatkṛtam ||4||
ātmāagnihotravahnau tu prāṇāyāmairvivardhite |
viśuddhacittahaviṣā vidhyuktaṁ karma juhvataḥ ||5||
niṣkṛtistasya kiṁ bāle kṛtakṛtyastadā khalu |
viyoge sati samprāpte jīvātmaparamātmanoḥ ||6||

Thus spoken to by one who enquires into the Brahman (Gārgī), Yājñavalkya, the greatest among men, who has realized the Brahman, looked at her and said as follows.

Yājñavalkya said:

For the person who is absorbed in yoga (samādhi) that which must be done at the two sandhis or at night, is done (completed) by yoga (samādhi) itself, beautiful [Gārgī]! Gārgī, how can there be any purification for one who fulfills his duties by offering his pure mind in the holy fire of the self, which is kindled by the practice of prāṇāyāma? He is then one who has done everything that is to be done, is he not?

7-10: When not in a state of yoga (samādhi), even a realized person must do all the Vedic duties.

vidhyuktaṁ karma kartavyaṁ brahmavidbhiśca nityaśaḥ |
viyogakāle yogī ca duḥkhamityeva yastyajet ||7||
karmāṇi tasya nilayaḥ nirayaḥ parikīrtitaḥ |
na dehināṁ yataḥ śakyaṁ tyaktuṁ karmāṇyaśeṣataḥ ||8||
tasmādāmaraṇādvaidhaṁ kartavyaṁ yogibhiḥ sadā |
tvaṁ caiva mātyayā gārgi vaidhaṁ karma samācara ||9||
yogena paramātmānaṁ yajaṁstyaja kalevaram |

When there is a separation between the self and the Divine, the actions laid down in the Vedas must be done, even by those who have realized the Brahman. At that time of separation (when not in samādhi), the yogi who gives up these actions thinking that they cause discomfort, his dwelling place will be one of suffering.

No one who has (is identified with) a body (no living being) can ever give up actions completely. Therefore, the actions prescribed by the Vedas should be performed by all yogis always until the time of death. Gārgī, you too must not slip. Perform all the actions said by the Vedas. Worshipping the Divine, through the practice of yoga, give up your body.

10-12: Instruction to Gārgī to attain freedom through the practice of yoga. Yājñavalkya's request to all the sages to return to their respective hermitages.

ityevamuktvā bhagavānyājñavalkyastaponidhiḥ ||10||
ṛśīnālokya netrābhyāṁ vākyametadabhāṣata |
sandhyāmupāsya vidhivatpaścimāṁ susamāhitāḥ ||11||
gacchantu sāmpratam sarve ṛṣayaḥ svāśramaṁ prati |
ityevamuktā muninā munayaḥ saṁśritavratāḥ ||12||

Having spoken thus, Yājñavalkya, the one fit to be worshipped, the repository of austerity, looked at the sages and spoke [again] as follows: "Having performed in the proper manner the daily ritual to be done in the evening, with a focused mind, let all the sages now proceed to their hermitages."

13-16: The sages return to their respective hermitages, after duly saluting Yājñavalkya.

viśvāmitro vasiṣṭhaśca gautamaścāṅgirāstathā |
agastyo nāradaścaiva vālmīkirbādarāyaṇiḥ ||13||
paiṅgidīrghatamā vyāsaḥ śaunakaśca tapodhanaḥ |
bhārgavaḥ kāśyapaścaiva bharadvājastathaiva ca ||14||
tapasvinastathā cānye vedavedāṅgavedinaḥ |
yājñavalkyaṁ susampūjya gīrbhirāśīrbhiruttamaiḥ ||15||
te yānti munayaḥ sarve svāśrameṣu yathāgatam |

Having thus been told by the sage [Yājñavalkya], the sages, Viśvāmitra, Vasiṣṭha, Gautama, Aṅgira, Agastya, Nārada, Vālmīki, Śuka, Paiṅgidīrghatama, Vyāsa, Śaunaka, Bhārgava, Kāśyapa, Bharadvāja and others who are absorbed in their austerities, who have known the essence of the Vedas and the vedāṅgas, having worshipped Yājñavalkya in a befitting manner, with auspicious chants [from the Vedas], return to their respective hermitages in the manner they arrived.

16-19: Gārgī's request to Yājñavalkya to explain the whole of yoga with all its eight limbs concisely.

gateṣu svāśrameṣveṣu tāpaseṣu tapodhanā ||16||
praṇamya daṇḍavadbhūmau vākyametadabhāṣata |
gārgyuvāca--
bhagavansarvaśāstrajña sarvabhūtahite rata ||17||
bhavamokṣāya yogīndra bhavadbhirbhāṣitam tu yat |
yamādyaṣṭāṅgasahito yogo muktestu sādhanam ||18||
tadetadvismṛtam sarvaṁ sarvajñaṁ tava sannidhau |
yogaṁ mamopadiśyādya sāṅgaṁ saṅkṣeparūpataḥ ||19||
trāatumarhasi sarvajña janmasaṁsārasāgarāt |

When the sages returned to their respective hermitages, [Gārgī], rich in austerity, prostrated on the ground like a stick and spoke as follows. Gārgī said, "Bhagavān![88] One who has realized all the scriptures, who is interested in the welfare of all beings, the foremost among the yogis! The yoga with eight limbs, starting from yama, which was explained by you as a means for freedom, has been completely forgotten [by me] in your presence itself. Therefore, all knowing [Yājñavalkya]! Protect me from the ocean of birth and bondage by explaining to me yoga with its limbs in a concise form."

20-22: Yājñavalkya's consent to explain the path of yoga concisely.

ityukto brahmavādinyā brahmavidbrāhmaṇastadā ||20||
ālokya kṛpayā dīnāṁ smitapūrvamabhāṣata |
uttiṣṭhottiṣṭha kiṁ śeṣe bhūmau gārgi varānane ||21||
vakṣyāmi te samāsena yogaṁ samprati taṁ śṛṇu ||22||
iti śrīyogayājñavalkye ekādaśo'dhyāyaḥ ||

Having thus been told by [Gārgī], who is desirous of realizing the Brahman, the one who has realized the Brahman [Yājñavalkya], looking at

---

[88] The word "Bhagavān" is usually used to address one who has attained freedom.

the humble Gārgī and smiling benevolently, said, "Arise beautiful Gārgī! Why do you prostrate thus on the ground? I shall now explain yoga to you concisely. Listen to it."

Chapter XII

OUTLINE

This single chapter contains the essence of the entire book. Yājñavalkya explains here the yogic path to freedom, in a concise manner. For the purpose of understanding, the verses can be divided into sections describing seven stages of progression along this path.

1-7: First stage: kindling of the agni by prāṇa.

8-13: Second stage: awakening of kuṇḍalinī.

14-20: Third stage: movement of the prāṇa to the heart-lotus, through the suṣumnā nāḍī.

21: Fourth stage: further ascent of prāṇa.

22-26: Fifth stage: the focusing of prāṇa in the center of the eyebrows.

27-29: Sixth stage: continued absorption of the mind and prāṇa in the center of the eyebrows—the abode of Viṣṇu.

30-35: Seventh stage: attainment of freedom.

36-40: The benefits of such yoga practice.

41: Importance of daily duties (nityakarma) along with the practice of yoga.

42: Yājñavalkya enters into solitude in samādhi after explaining the greatest secret.

43-44: Gārgī worships Yājñavalkya, having understood the essence of yoga and recedes into solitude with complete happiness.

45: Praise of Vāsudeva, the Divine.

46: Yājñavalkya and Gārgī are always present, beholding the Divine in themselves.

Chapter XII

1-7: First stage: kindling of the agni by prāṇa.

savyena gulphena gudam nipīḍya savyetareṇaiva nipīḍya sandhim |
savyetaraṁ nyasya karetarasminśikhāṁ samālokaya pāvakasya ||1||
āyurvidhātakṛtprāṇo niruddhastvāsanena vai |
yāti gārgi tadāpānat kulaṁ vahneḥ śanaiḥ śanaiḥ ||2||
vāyunā vātito vahnirapānena śanaiḥ śanaiḥ |
tato jvalati sarveṣāṁ svakule dehamadhyame ||3||
prātaḥkāle pradoṣe ca niśīthe ca samāhitaḥ |
muhūrtamabhyasedevam yāvat pañcadinadvayam ||4||
tatasvātmani viprendre pratyayāśca pṛthakpṛthak |
sambhavanti tadā tasya jito yena samīraṇaḥ ||5||
śarīralaghutā dīptirvahnerjaṭharavartinaḥ |
nādābhivyaktirityete cihnānyādau bhavanti hi ||6||
alpamūtrapurīṣaḥ syātṣaṇmāse vatsare'pi vā |
āsane vāhane paścānna bhetavyaṁ trivatsarāt ||7||

Yājñavalkya said:

Pressing the anus with the left ankle and the perineum with the right ankle, placing the right palm on the left, see (meditate on) the flames of the fire. Then, the prāṇa which reduces the life span [when it is dispersed], is blocked and slowly moves from bottom (apāna) to the abode of fire, Gārgī. The fire which is fanned slowly by the apāna vāyu glows in its abode in the center of the body (dehamadhya), in all beings.

In the morning, evening and midnight, with a focused and balanced mind, one should practice this for ten days for a duration of ninety minutes (1 muhūrta).

Illustrious [Gārgī]! Various experiences then arise in one who has conquered the prāṇa. Lightness in the body, brightness of the abdominal fire (improved digestion and metabolism), and appearance of nāda are the first indications. In six months or one year, there is reduction of the urine and stools, and after three years, one overcomes fear.

8-13: Second stage: awakening of kuṇḍalinī.

tato'nilaṁ vāyusakhena sārdhaṁ dhiyā samāropya nirodhayettam |
dhyāyansadā cakriṇamaprabuddham nābhau sadā kuṇḍalinīniviṣṭam ||8||
śirāṁ samāveṣya mukhena madhyāmanyāśca bhogena śirāstathaiva |
svapucchamāsyena nigṛhya samyakpathaśca saṁyamya marudgaṇānām ||9||
prasuptanāgendravaducchavasantī sadā prabuddhā prabhayā jvalantī |
nābhau sadā tiṣṭhati kuṇḍalī sā tiryaksu deheṣu tathetareṣu ||10||
vāyunā vihṛtavahniśikhābhiḥ kandamadhyagatanaḍīṣu samsthām |
kuṇḍalīṁ dahati yastvahirūpām saṁsmarannaravarastu sa eva ||11||
santaptā vahninā tatra vāyunā ca pracālitā |
prasārya phaṇabhṛdbhogaṁ prabodham yāti sā tadā ||12||
bodhaṁ gate cakriṇi nābhimadhye prāṇāḥ susambhūya kalevare'smin |
caranti sarve saha vahninaiva yathā paṭe tantugatistathaiva ||13||

Then, drawing the prāṇa inside, along with the fire, using the mind, focus it in the unawakened kuṇḍalinī, in the navel. Covering the suṣumnā by her mouth and the other nāḍīs by her hood, holding her own tail by her mouth, blocking the path of the prāṇa, breathing like a sleeping snake, yet always awake, shining by her own luster, the kuṇḍalinī resides always in the navel region (nābhi) in the bodies of all beings.

The one who, with total concentration, burns the kuṇḍalinī, which is in the form of a snake in the nāḍīs in the middle of the kandasthāna (which blocks the flow of prāṇa in the nāḍīs), by the flames of the fire which are fanned by the prāṇa, is the most illustrious among men.

Kuṇḍalinī, in the form of a snake, burnt by the fire, and shaken/moved by the vāyu, spreads her hood and awakens. When the kuṇḍalinī in the center of the navel region (nābhi) is awakened, the vāyus in the body join together and move [unitedly], along with the fire, like the strands of thread in a cloth.

14-20: Third stage: movement of the prāṇa to the heart-lotus, through the suṣumnā nāḍī.

jitvaivam cakriṇaḥ sthānaṁ sadā dhyānaparāyaṇaḥ |
tato nayedapānaṁ to nābherūrdhvamidaṁ smaran ||14||
vāyuryathā vāyusakhena sārdhaṁ nābhiṁ tvatikramya gataḥ śarīre |
rogāśca naśyanti balābhivṛddhiḥ kāntistadānīmabhavatprabuddhe ||15||
brahmarandhramukhamatra vāyavaḥ pāvakena saha yānti samūhya |
kenacidiha vadāmi tavāhaṁ vīkṣaṇād hṛdi sudīpaśikhāyāḥ ||16||
nirodhitaḥ syādhṛdi tena vāyuḥ madhye yadā vāyusakhena sārdham |
sahasrapatrasya mukhaṁ praviśya kuryātpunastūrdhvamukhaṁ dvijendre ||17||
prabuddhahṛdayāmbhoje gārgyasminbrahmaṇaḥ pure |
bālārkaśreṇivadvyomni virarāja samīraṇaḥ ||18||
hṛnmadhyāttu suṣumnāyāṁ saṁsthito hutabhuktadā |
sajalāmbudamālāsu vidyullekheva rājate ||19||
prabuddhahṛtpadmani saṁsthitegnau prāṇe ca tasminviniveśite ca |
cihnāni bāhyāni tathāntarāṇi dīpādi dṛśyāṇi bhavanti tasya ||20||

Having thus conquered the seat of the kunḍalinī, always absorbed in dhyāna, one must lead the apāna vāyu towards the region above the navel (nābhi). When the prāṇa along with the fire in the body moves beyond the navel (nābhi), all diseases are destroyed, strength increases, and the body becomes lustrous. Now the vāyus, joining together, along with the fire, move to the opening in the crown of the head (brahmarandhra).

I shall tell you a means for this. [The means is] seeing (meditating on) the bright flames [of the fire] in the heart. By this, when the vāyu along with the agni is stopped in the center of the heart, it enters the opening of the thousand-petalled heart-lotus and must be made to face (move) upwards again

Gārgī, in this abode of the Brahman (in this body), in the fully-blossomed lotus of the heart, the prāṇa shines in that space like the rising sun. Then the fire shines like a streak of lightning in a range of clouds, from the center of the heart in the suṣumnā. When the fire is established in the bloomed (awakened) heart-lotus and the prāṇa has been made to enter into it, various signs, both external and internal, come about, [for instance,] like the vision of a flame.

21: Fourth stage: further ascent of prāṇa.

vāyumunnaya tatastu savahniṁ vyāharanpraṇavamatra sabinduṁ |
bālacandrasadṛśe tu lalāṭe bālacandramavalokaya buddhyā ||21||

Then, raising the prāṇa along with the fire, reciting the praṇava, meditate upon the disc of the rising moon in the forehead.

22-26: Fifth stage: the focusing of prāṇa in the center of the eyebrows.

savahniṁ vāyumāropya bhruvormadhye dhiyā tadā |
dhyāyedananyadhīḥ paścādantarātmānamantare ||22||
madhyame'pi hṛdaye ca lalāṭe sthāṇuvajjvalati liṅgamadṛśyam |
asti gārgi paramārthamidaṁ tvaṁ paśya paśya manasā rucirūpam ||23||
lalāṭamadhye hṛdayāmbuje ca yaḥ paśyati jñāmayīṁ prabhāṁ tu |
śaktiṁ sadā dīpavadujjvalantīṁ sa paśyati brahmavidekādṛṣṭyā ||24||
mano layam yadā yāti bhrūmadhye yogināṁ nṛṇām |
jihvāmūle'mṛtasrāvo bhrūmadhye cātmadarśanam ||25||
kampanaṁ ca tathā mūrdhno manasaivātmadarśanaṁ |
devodyānāni ramyāṇi nakṣatrāṇi ca candramāḥ |
ṛṣayaḥ siddhagandharvāḥ prakāśaṁ yānti yoginām ||26||

Then, drawing and holding the prāṇa along with the fire at the center of the eyebrows, mentally, with total concentration, one must meditate on one's self within. In the middle of the body, the heart and the forehead, like a pillar, shines an imperceptible liṅga. This is truly the greatest to be attained, Gārgī. You too behold that beautiful form with your mind.

The one who sees with an unfaltering gaze, in the center of the forehead and the heart-lotus, the glow that shines like a lamp, which is the embodiment of knowledge and power—he is the one who has realized the Brahman.

When the mind of the yogi is totally absorbed in the center of the eyebrows, then nectar flows from the base of the tongue, and the self is seen at the center of the eyebrows. A trembling [sensation] of the head, the perception of the self through the mind, beautiful celestial gardens, stars and the moon, the ṛṣis, siddhas, and gandharvas (sages and celestial beings) all appear to the yogis.

27-29: Sixth stage: continued absorption of the mind and prāṇa in the center of the eyebrows—the abode of Viṣṇu.

bhruvontare viṣṇupade ṛcau tu mano layam yāvadiyātprabuddhe |
tāvatsamabhyasya punaḥ khamadhye sukham sadā saṁsmara pūrṇarūpam ||27||
samīraṇe viṣṇupade niviṣṭe jīve ca tasminnamṛte ca saṁsthe |
tasminstadā yāti mano layaṁ cenmukteḥ samīpaṁ taditi bruvanti ||28||
samīraṇe viṣṇupade niviṣṭe viśuddhabuddhau ca tadātmaniṣṭhe |
ānandamatyadbhutamasti satyaṁ tvaṁ gārgi paśyādya viśuddhabuddhyā ||29||

Practice this till the mind is absorbed in the center of the eyebrows, in the abode of Viṣṇu, and then again meditate in that space on that which is complete, and which is the embodiment of bliss. When the prāṇa has reached the abode of Viṣṇu, and the self is established in that bliss, if the mind becomes absorbed, that leads to a state very close to freedom.

When the prāṇa has reached the abode of Viṣṇu, and when the mind is clear and established in the self, there is indescribable bliss. Gārgī! Behold it now with a clear mind.

30-35: Seventh stage: attainment of freedom.

evaṁ samabhyasya sudīrghakālaṁ yamādibhiryuktatanurmitāśīḥ |
ātmānamāsādya guhāṁ praviṣṭaṁ muktiṁ vraja brahmapure punastvam ||30||
bhūtāni yasmātprabhavanti gārgi yenaiva jīvanti carācarāṇi |
jātāni yasminvilayaṁ prayānti tadbrahma viddhīti vadanti sarve ||31||

hṛtpaṅkaje vyomni yadekarūpaṁ satyaṁ sadānandamayaṁ susūkṣmam |
tadbrahma nirbhāsamayaṁ guhāyāmiti śrutiśceti samāmananti ||32||
aṇoraṇīyānmahato mahīyānātmā guhāyaṁ nihito'sya jantoḥ |
tamakratuṁ paśya viśuddhabuddhyā prayāṇakāle ca vihīnaśokā ||33||
prabhañjanaṁ mūrdhnigataṁ savahniṁ dhiyā samāsādya gurūpadeśāt |
mūrdhānamudbhidya punaḥ khamadhye
prāṇāstyajoṅkāaramanusmaraṁstvam ||34||
īpsayā yadi śarīravisargaṁ jñātumiccasi sakhe tava vakṣye |
vyāharanpraṇavamunnaya mūrdhni bhidya yojaya tamātmanikāyam ||35||

Having practiced thus for a long time, with a regulated food intake, observing yama and the other limbs, having realized the self which is in the cave/recess, attain freedom in this abode of the Brahman (in this body).

That from which all beings originate, by which (whose support) everything, living and non-living, is sustained, and into which [all the above] dissolve, know that to be the Brahman. So says all [who have realized the Brahman].

That which is one, true, always the personification of bliss, very subtle, the epitome of effulgence, present in a cave, in the space of the heart-lotus, that is the Brahman. Thus say the Vedas too.

The subtlest of the subtle, the greatest of the great, the self is present in the internal space of all beings. See that [self], which is devoid of desire, at the time of death, without sorrow, with a clear mind.

Having controlled the prāṇa, which has reached the crown of the head along with the fire, using the intellect, by initiation from one's guru, meditating on OM, split open the crown of the head and give up the prāṇa in that space.

My friend,[89] if you wish to know how to leave the body as per your wish, I will tell you. Reciting the praṇava mentally, drawing the prāṇa to the crown of the head, splitting [the crown of the head], unite it (the prāṇa) with the self.

36-40: The benefits of such yoga practice.

etatpavitraṁ paramaṁ yogamaṣṭāṅgasaṁyutam |
jñānaṁ guhyatamaṁ puṇyaṁ kīrtitaṁ te varānane ||36||
ya idam śṛṇuyānnityaṁ yogākhyānaṁ narottamaḥ |
sarvapāpavinirmuktaḥ samyagjñānī bhaviṣyati ||37||
yastvetatcchrāvayedvidvānnityaṁ bhaktisamanvitaḥ |
ekajanmakṛtaṁ pāpaṁ dinenaikena naśyati ||38||
śṛṇuyādyaḥ sakṛdvāpi yogākhyānamidaṁ naraḥ |
ajñānajanitaṁ pāpaṁ sarvaṁ tasya praṇaśyati ||39||
anutiṣṭhanti ye nityamātmajñānasamanvitam |
nityakarmāṇi tāndṛṣṭvā devāśca praṇamanti hi ||40||

Yoga with its eight limbs, which is holy, the purest, greatest and most secret among all knowledge, has been explained to you, beautiful [Gārgī]. The illustrious one who always listens to (and practices according to) this exposition of yoga is freed from all bondage and will become a realized person. In the learned person, who expounds this [yoga] always, with devotion and reverence, all bondage caused in one lifetime is destroyed in one day. All bondage caused due to ignorance perishes in the person who listens to this exposition on yoga even once. Even the celestials bow on seeing the ones who always perform all their daily duties [in accordance with the Vedas] along with realization of the self.

---

[89] Here Yājñavalkya addresses his wife, Gārgī, as "sakhā" meaning "my friend." A wife is considered the best friend of her husband and vice versa. The same sentiment is echoed in the sections of the Vedas which speak of the rituals for marriage. Śaṅkarācārya also says, "The wife is the best friend of the husband."

41: Importance of daily duties (nityakarma) along with the practice of yoga.

tasmājjñānena dehāntaṁ nityaṁ karma yathāvadhi |
kartavyaṁ dehibhirgārgi yogaśca bhavabhīrubhiḥ ||41||

Therefore, as long as one lives, daily duties (in accordance with the Vedas) along with jñāna (spiritual realization or non-attachment), and yoga too must be done in the prescribed manner by all beings who fear bondage.

42: Yājñavalkya enters into solitude in samādhi after explaining the greatest secret.

ityevamuktvā bhagavānrahasye rahasyajaṁ muktikaraṁ tu tuasyāḥ |
yogāmṛtaṁ bandhavināśahetuṁ samādhimāste rahasi dvijendraḥ ||42||

Having thus explained in solitude, the nectar of yoga, which was born in solitude (through secluded practice), which is the cause for destruction of all bondage and leads to freedom, to her [Gārgī], [Yājñavalkya], the one fit to be worshipped, greatest among brahmins, entered into samādhi in solitude.

43-44: Gārgī worships Yājñavalkya, having understood the essence of yoga and recedes into solitude with complete happiness.

sa taṁ tu sampūjya muniṁ bruvantaṁ vidyānidhiṁ brahmavidāṁ variṣṭham |
gīrbhiḥ praṇāmaiśca satāṁ variṣṭhaṁ sadā mudam prāpa varāṁ viśuddhām ||43||
yogaṁ susaṅgṛhya tadā rahasye rahasyajaṁ muktikaraṁ ca jantoḥ |
samsāramutsṛjya sadā mudānvitā vane rahasyāvasathe viveśa ||44||

Having worshipped with chants and prostrations the sage (Yājñavalkya) who had spoken thus, and is the storehouse of all learning, the greatest among the ones who have realized the Brahman, the greatest among seers, [Gārgī] attained the greatest and purest happiness.

Then, in solitude, having clearly understood yoga which is born in solitude, and is the cause for freedom of all beings, having given up worldly bondage, [Gārgī] entered a solitary place in the forest with complete happiness.

45: Praise of Vāsudeva, the Divine.

yena prapañcaṁ paripūrṇametadyenaiva viśvaṁ pratibhāti sarvam |
taṁ vāsudevaṁ śrutimūrdhni jātaṁ paśyansadāste hṛdi mūrdhni cānvaham ||45||

[Thus] she remained, always seeing (meditating on) in the crown of the head and in the heart, that Vāsudeva (the Divine), spoken of by the Vedas, by whom this entire world is complete and radiant.

46: Yājñavalkya and Gārgī are always present, beholding the Divine in themselves.

yadekamavyaktamanantamacyutaṁ prapañcajanmādikṛdaprameyam |
taṁ vāsudevaṁ śrutimūrdhni jātaṁ paśyansadāste hṛdi mūrdhni cānvaham ||46||
iti śrīyogayājñavalkye dvādaśo'dhyāyaḥ ||
samāptamidaṁ yogaśāstram ||

Seeing (meditating on) always in the heart and the crown of the head, that Vāsudeva, who is one, immeasurable, unmanifest, endless, beyond change, responsible for the creation, sustenance and destruction of the world, Yājñavalkya and Gārgī are always present.

Appendix I: Comparisons of Versions

The BBRA publication has 504 verses. The Trivandrum/KYM publication misses 33 full verses and 13 half verses for a total of 464½ verses. Below we summarize the differences between the BBRA/this publication and the Trivandrum/KYM publications. The abbreviations "i" and "ii" indicate the first and second lines of a verse, respectively. For example, "57/i" refers to the first line of verse 57. If "i" or "ii" are not specified, the whole verse is missing.

Chapter	Number of verses		Missing verses in Trivandrum/KYM Publication
	BBRA	Trivandrum/KYM	
1	70	68½	37, 57/i
2	19	19	-
3	18	18	-
4	71½	70½	53
5	22	21	3/i, 16/i
6	92	80	7/ii, 56/ii, 62, 10 verses in appendix
7	37	30	5, 6, 7, 9, 10/i, 19/ii, 25, 26
8	39½	23	1/ii, 4/ii, 11/ii, 12, 13, 14, 15, 16, 17, 18, 19, 20, 21, 22, 23, 24, 25, 37/ii, 38/i
9	44	44	-
10	23½	23	18/i
11	21½	21½	-
12	46	46	-
Total	504	464½	33 full verses and 13 half verses

Appendix II: Devanagari Text

प्रथमोऽध्यायः

याज्ञवल्क्यं मुनिश्रेष्ठं सर्वज्ञं ज्ञाननिर्मलम्।

सर्वशास्त्रार्थतत्वज्ञं सदा ध्यानपरायणम्॥ १॥

वेदवेदाङ्गतत्वज्ञं योगेषु परिनिष्ठितम्।

जितेन्द्रियं जितक्रोधं जिताहारं जितामयम्॥ २॥

तपस्विनं जितामित्रं ब्रह्मण्यं ब्राह्मणप्रियम्।

तपोवनगतं सौम्यं सन्ध्योपासनतत्परम्॥ ३॥

ब्रह्मविद्भिर्महाभागैर्ब्राह्मणैश्च समावृतम्।

सर्वभूतसमं शान्तं सत्यसन्धं गतक्लमम्॥ ४॥

गुणज्ञं सर्वभूतेषु परार्थैकप्रयोजनम्।

ब्रुवन्तं परमात्मानमृषीणामुग्रतेजसाम्॥ ५॥

तमेवं गुणसंपन्नं नारीणामुत्तमा वधूः।

मैत्रेयी च महाभागा गार्गी च ब्रह्मविद्वरा॥ ६॥

सभामध्यगता चेयमृषीणामुग्रतेजसाम्।

प्रणम्य दण्डवद्भूमौ गार्ग्यैतद्वाक्यमब्रवीत्॥ ७॥

गार्ग्युवाच--

भगवन्सर्वशास्त्रज्ञ सर्वभूतहिते रत।

योगतत्वं मम ब्रूहि साङ्गोपाङ्गं विधानतः॥ ८॥

एवं पृष्टः स भगवान्सभामध्ये स्त्रिया तया।

ऋषीनालोक्य नेत्राभ्यां वाक्यमेतदभाषत॥ ।९॥

याज्ञवल्क्य उवाच--

उत्तिष्ठोत्तिष्ठ भद्रं ते गार्गि ब्रह्मविदां वरे।

वक्ष्यामि योगसर्वस्वं ब्रह्मणा कीर्तितं पुरा॥ १०॥

समाहितमना गार्गि श‍ृणु त्वं गदतो मम।

इत्युक्त्वा ब्रह्मविच्छ्रेष्ठो याज्ञवल्क्यस्तपोनिधिः॥ ११॥

नारायणं जगन्नाथं सर्वभूतहृदि स्थितम्।

वासुदेवं जगद्योनिं योगिध्येयं निरञ्जनम्॥ १२॥

आनन्दममृतं नित्यं परमात्मानमीश्वरम्।

ध्यायन्हृदि हृषीकेशं मनसा सुसमाहितः॥ १३॥

नेत्राभ्यां तां समलोक्य कृपया वाक्यमब्रवीत्।

एह्येहि गार्गि सर्वज्ञे सर्वशास्त्रविशारदे॥ १४॥

योगं वक्ष्यामि विधिवद्धात्रोक्तं परमेष्ठिना।

मुनयः श्रूयतामत्र गार्ग्या सह समाहिताः॥ १५॥

पद्मासने समासीनं चतुराननमव्ययम्।

चराचराणां स्रष्टारं ब्रह्माणं परमेष्ठिनम्॥ १६॥

कदाचित्तत्र गत्वाहं स्तुत्वा स्तोत्रैः प्रणम्य च।

पृष्टवानिममेवार्थं यन्मां त्वं परिपृच्छसि॥ १७॥

देवदेव जगन्नाथ चतुर्मुख पितामह।

येनाहं यामि निर्वाणं कर्मणा मोक्षमव्ययम्॥ १८॥

ज्ञानं च परमं गुह्यं यथावद्ब्रूहि मे प्रभो।

मयैवमुक्तो द्रुहिणः स्वयंभूर्लोकनायकः॥ १९॥

मामालोक्य प्रसन्नात्मा ज्ञानकर्माण्यभाषत।

ज्ञानस्य द्विविधौ ज्ञेयौ पन्थानौ वेदचोदितौ॥ २०॥

अनुष्ठितौ तौ विद्वद्भिः प्रवर्तकनिवर्तकौ।
वर्णाश्रमोक्तं यत्कर्म कामसङ्कल्पपुर्वकम्॥ २१॥

प्रवर्तकं भवेदेतत्पुनरावृत्तिहेतुकम्।
कर्तव्यमिति विध्युक्तं कर्म कामविवर्जितम्॥ २२॥

येन यत्क्रियते सम्यक् ज्ञानयुक्तं निवर्तकम्।
निवर्तकं हि पुरुषं निवर्तयति जन्मतः॥ २३॥

प्रवर्तकं हि सर्वत्र पुनरावृत्तिहेतुकम्।
वर्णाश्रमोक्तं कर्मैव विध्युक्तं कामवर्जितम्॥ २४॥

विधिवत्कुर्वतस्तस्य मुक्तिर्गार्गि करे स्थिता।
वर्णाश्रमोक्तं कर्मैव विधिवत्कामपूर्वकम्॥ २५॥

येन यत्क्रियते तस्य गर्भवासः करे स्थितः।
संसारभीरुभिस्तस्मात्विध्युक्तं कामवर्जितम्॥ २६॥

विधिवत् कर्म कर्तव्यं ज्ञानेन सह सर्वदा।
जाताश्च त्रिषु लोकेषु आनुलोम्येन मानवाः॥ २७॥

ते देवानामृषीणां च पितृणामृणिनस्तथा।
ऋषिभ्यो ब्रह्मचर्येण पितृभ्यश्च सुतैस्तथा॥ २८॥

कुर्याद्यज्ञेन देवेभ्यः स्वाश्रमं धर्ममाचरन्।
चत्वारो ब्राह्मणस्योक्ता आश्रमाः श्रुतिचोदिताः॥ २९॥

क्षत्रियस्य त्रयः प्रोक्ता द्वावेकौ वैश्यशूद्रयोः।
अधीत्य वेदं वेदार्थं साङ्गोपाङ्गं विधानतः॥ ३०॥

स्नायाद्विध्युक्तमार्गेण ब्रह्मचर्यव्रतं चरन्।
संस्कृतायां सवर्णायां पुत्रमुत्पादयेत्ततः॥ ३१॥

यजेदग्नौ तु विधिवत्भार्यया सह वा विना।

कान्तारे विजने देशे फलमूलोदकान्विते॥ ३२॥

तपश्चरन्वसेन्नित्यं साग्निहोत्रः समाहितः।

आत्मन्यग्नीन्समारोप्य सन्न्यसेद्विधिना ततः॥ ३३॥

सन्यासाश्रमसंयुक्तो नित्यं कर्म समाचरन्।

यावत्क्षेत्री भवेत्तावत् यजेदात्मानमात्मनि॥ ३४॥

क्षत्रियश्च चरेदेवमासन्यासाश्रमात्सदा।

वानप्रस्थाश्रमादेवं चरेद्वैश्यः समाहितः॥ ३५॥

शूद्रः शुश्रूषया नित्यं गृहस्थाश्रमं आचरेत्।

शूद्रस्य ब्रह्मचर्यं च मुनिभिः कैश्चिदिष्यते॥ ३६॥

आनुलोम्यप्रसूतानां त्रयाणामाश्रमास्त्रयः।

शूद्रवच्छूद्रजातानां आचारः कीर्तितो बुधैः॥ ३७॥

चतुर्णामाश्रमस्थानामहन्यहनि नित्यशः।

विध्युक्तं कर्म कर्तव्यं कामसङ्कल्पवर्जितम्॥ ३८॥

तस्मात्त्वमपि योगीन्द्र स्वाश्रमं धर्ममाचरन्।

श्रद्धया विधिवत्सम्यक् ज्ञानकर्म समाचर॥ ३९॥

इति मे कर्मसर्वस्वं योगरूपं च तत्वतः।

उपदिश्य ततो ब्रह्मा योगनिष्ठोऽभवत्स्वयम्॥ ४०॥

श्रुत्वैतद्याज्ञवल्क्योक्तं वाक्यं गार्गी मुदान्विता।

पुनः प्राह मुनिश्रेष्ठमृषीमध्ये वरानना॥ ४१॥

गार्ग्युवाच --

ज्ञानेन सह योगीन्द्र विध्युक्तं कर्म कुर्वतः।

त्वयोक्तं मुक्तिरस्तीति तयोर्ज्ञानं वद प्रभो॥ ४२॥

भार्यया त्वेवमुक्तस्तु याज्ञवल्क्यस्तपोनिधिः।

तां समालोक्य कृपया ज्ञानरूपमभाषत॥ ४३॥

याज्ञवल्क्य उवाच--

ज्ञानं योगात्मकं विद्धि योगश्चाष्टाङ्गसंयुतः।

संयोगो योग इत्युक्तो जीवात्मपरमात्मनोः॥ ४४॥

वक्ष्याम्यङ्गानि ते सम्यग्यथा पूर्वं मया श्रुतम्।

समाहितमना गार्गी ऋषिभिः सह संश्रृणु॥ ४५॥

यमश्च नियमश्चैव आसनं च तथैव च।

प्राणायामस्तथा गार्गी प्रत्याहारश्च धारणा॥ ४६॥

ध्यानं समाधिरेतानि योगाङ्गानि वरानने।

यमस्च नियमश्चैव दशधा संप्रकीर्तितः॥ ४७॥

आसनान्युत्तमान्यष्टौ त्रयं तेषूत्तमोत्तमम्।

प्राणयामस्त्रिधा प्रोक्तः प्रत्यहारश्च पञ्चधा॥ ४८॥

धारणा पञ्चधा प्रोक्ता ध्यानं षोढा प्रकीर्तितम्।

त्रयं तेषूत्तमं प्रोक्तं समाधिस्त्वेकरूपकः॥ ४९॥

बहुधा केचिदिच्छन्ति विस्तरेण पृथक् श्रृणु।

अहिंसा सत्यमस्तेयं ब्रह्मचर्यं दयार्जवम्॥ ५०॥

क्षमाधृतिर्मिताहारः शौचं त्वेते यमा दश।

कर्मणा मनसा वाचा सर्वभूतेषु सर्वदा॥ ५१॥

अक्लेशजननं प्रोक्तमहिंसात्वेन योगिभिः।

विध्युक्तं चेदहिंसा स्यात्क्लेशजन्मैव जन्तुषु॥ ५२॥

वेदेनोक्तेऽपि हिंसास्यादभिचारादि कर्म यत्।

सत्यं भूतहितं प्रोक्तं न यथार्थाभिभाषणम्॥ ५३॥

कर्मणा मनसा वाचा परद्रव्येषु निःस्पृहा।

अस्तेयमिति सा प्रोक्ता ऋषिभिस्तत्त्वदर्शिभिः॥ ५४॥

कर्मणा मनसा वाचा सर्वावस्थासु सर्वदा।

सर्वत्र मैथुनत्यागो ब्रह्मचर्यं प्रचक्षते॥ ५५॥

ब्रह्मचर्याश्रमस्थानां यतीनां नैष्ठिकस्य च।

ब्रह्मचर्यं तु तत्प्रोक्तं तथैवारण्यवासिनाम्॥ ५६॥

ऋतावृतौ स्वदारेषु सङ्गतिर्या विधानतः।

ब्रह्मचर्यं तु तत्प्रोक्तं गृहस्थाश्रमवासिनाम्॥ ५७॥

राज्ञश्चैव गृहस्थस्य ब्रह्मचर्यं प्रकीर्तितम्।

विशां वृत्तवतां चैव केचिदिच्छन्ति पण्डिताः॥ ५८॥

शुश्रूषैव तु शूद्रस्य ब्रह्मचर्यं प्रकीर्तितम्।

शुश्रूषा वा गुरोर्नित्यं ब्रह्मचर्यमुदाहृतम्॥ ५९॥

गुरवः पञ्च सर्वेषां चतुर्णां श्रुतिचोदिताः।

माता पिता तथाचार्यो मातुलः श्वशुरस्तथा॥ ६०॥

एषु मुख्यास्त्रयः प्रोक्ता आचार्यः पितरौ तथा।

एषु मुख्यतमस्त्वेक आचार्यः परमार्थवित्॥ ६१॥

तमेवं ब्रह्माविच्छ्रेष्ठं नित्यकर्मपरायणम्।

शुश्रूषयार्चयेन्नित्यं तुष्टोऽभूद्येन वा गुरुः॥ ६२॥

दया च सर्वभूतेषु सर्वत्रानुग्रहः स्मृतः।

विहितेषु तदन्येषु मनोवाक्कायकर्मणाम्॥ ६३॥

प्रवृत्तौ वा निवृत्तौ वा एकरूपत्वमार्जवम्।

प्रियाप्रियेषु सर्वेषु समत्वं यच्छरीरिणाम्॥ ६४॥

क्षमा सैवेति विद्वद्भिर्गदिता वेदवादिभिः।

अर्थहानौ च बन्धूनां वियोगेष्वपि सम्पदाम्॥ ६५॥

तयोः प्राप्तौ च सर्वत्र चित्तस्य स्थापनं धृतिः।

अष्टौ ग्रासा मुनेर्भक्ष्याः षोडशारण्यवासिनाम्॥ ६६॥

द्वात्रिंशच्च गृहस्थानां यथेष्टं ब्रह्मचारिणाम्।

एषामयं मिताहारो ह्यन्येषामल्पभोजनम्॥ ६७॥

शौचं तु द्विविधं प्रोक्तं बाह्यमाभ्यन्तरं तथा।

मृज्जलाभ्यां स्मृतं बाह्यं मनःशुद्धिस्तथान्तरम्॥ ६८॥

मनःशुद्धिश्च विज्ञेया धर्मेणाध्यात्मविद्यया।

आत्मविद्या च धर्मश्च पित्राचार्येण वानधे॥ ६९॥

तस्मात्सर्वेषु कालेषु सर्वैर्निःश्रेयसार्थिभिः।

गुरवः श्रुतसम्पन्ना मान्या वाङ्मनसादिभिः॥ ७०॥

इति श्रीयोगयाज्ञवल्क्ये प्रथमोऽध्यायः॥

द्वितीयोऽध्यायः

याज्ञवल्क्य उवाच--

तपः सन्तोष आस्तिक्यं दानमीश्वरपूजनम्।

सिद्धान्तश्रवणंचैव ह्रीर्मतिश्च जपो व्रतम्॥ १॥

एते तु नियमाः प्रोक्तास्तान्श्च सर्वान्पृथक् शृणु।

विधिनोक्तेन मार्गेण कृच्छ्रचान्द्रायनादिभिः॥ २॥

शरीरशोषणं प्राहुस्तापसास्तप उत्तमम्।

यदृच्छालाभतो नित्यमलं पुंसो भवेदिति॥ ३॥

या धीस्तामृषयः प्राहुः सन्तोषं सुखलक्षणम्।

धर्माधर्मेषु विश्वासो यस्तदास्तिक्यमुच्यते॥ ४॥

न्यायार्जितं धनं चान्नमन्यद्वा यत्प्रदीयते।

अर्थिभ्यः श्रद्धया युक्तं दानमेतदुदाहृतम्॥ ५॥

यत्प्रसन्नस्वभावेन विष्णुं वाऽप्यन्यमेव वा।

यथाशक्त्यर्चनं भक्त्या ह्येतदीश्वरपूजनम्॥ ६॥

रागाद्यपेतं हृदयं वागदुष्टानृतवादिना।

हिंसादिरहितः काय एतदीश्वरपूजनम्॥ ७॥

सिद्धान्तश्रवणं प्रोक्तं वेदान्तश्रवणं बुधैः।

द्विजवत्क्षत्रियस्योक्तं सिद्धान्तश्रवणं बुधैः॥ ८॥

विशां च केचिदिच्छन्ति शीलवृत्तवतां सताम्।

शूद्राणां च स्त्रियाश्चैव स्वधर्मस्थतपस्विनाम्॥ ९॥

सिद्धान्तश्रवणं प्रोक्तं पुराणश्रवणं बुधैः।

वेदलौकिकमार्गेषु कुत्सितं कर्म यद्भवेत्॥ १०॥

तस्मिन्भवति या लज्जा ह्रीस्तु सैवेति कीर्तिता।

विहितेषु च सर्वेषु श्रद्धा या सा मतिर्भवेत्॥ ११॥

गुरुणा चोपदिष्टोऽपि वेदबाह्यविवर्जितः।

विधिनोक्तेन मार्गेण मन्त्राभ्यासो जपः स्मृतः॥ १२॥

अधीत्य वेदं सूत्रं वा पुराणं सेतिहासकम्।

एतेष्वभ्यसनं यच्च तदभ्यासो जपः स्मृतः॥ १३॥

जपश्च द्विविधः प्रोक्तो वाचिको मानसस्तथा।

वाचिक उपांशुरुच्चैश्च द्विविधः परिकीर्तिततः॥ १४॥

मानसो मननध्यानभेदाद् द्वैविध्यमास्थितः।

उच्चैर्जपादुपांशुश्च सहस्रगुण उच्यते॥ १५॥

मानसस्तु तथोपांशोः सहस्रगुण उच्यते।

मानसाच्च तथा ध्यानं सहस्रगुणमुच्यते॥ १६॥

उच्चैर्जपस्तु सर्वेषां यथोक्तफलदो भवेत्।

नीचैः श्रुतो न चेत्सोऽपि श्रुतश्चेन्निष्फलो भवेत्॥ १७॥

ऋषिं छन्दोऽधिदैवं च ध्यायन्मन्त्रं च सर्वदा।

यस्तु मन्त्रजपो गार्गि स एव हि फलप्रदः॥ १८॥

प्रसन्नगुरुणा पूर्वमुपदिष्टं त्वनुज्ञया।

धर्मार्थमात्मसिद्ध्यर्थमुपायग्रहणं व्रतम्॥ १९॥

इति श्रीयोगयज्ञवल्क्ये द्वितीयोऽध्यायः।

तृतीयोऽध्यायः

याज्ञवल्क्य उवाच--

आसनान्यधुना वक्ष्ये श्रृणु गार्गि तपोधने।

स्वस्तिकं गोमुखं पद्मं वीरं सिंहासनं तथा॥ १॥

भद्रं मुक्तासनं चैव मयूरासनमेव च।

तथैतेषां वरारोहे पृथग्वक्ष्यामि लक्षणम्॥ २॥

जानोर्वोरन्तरे सम्यक्कृत्वा पादतले उभे।

ऋजुकायः सुखासीनः स्वस्तिकं तत्प्रचक्षते॥ ३॥

सीवन्यास्त्वात्मनः पार्श्वे गुल्फौ निक्षिप्य पादयोः।

सव्ये दक्षिणगुल्फं तु दक्षिणे दक्षिणेतरम्॥ ४॥

एतच्च स्वस्तिकं प्रोक्तं सर्वपापप्रणाशनम्।
सव्ये दक्षिणगुल्फं तु पृष्ठपार्श्वे नियोजयेत्॥५॥
दक्षिणेऽपि तथा सव्यं गोमुखं गोमुखं यथा।
अङ्गुष्ठौ च निबध्नीयाद्धस्ताभ्यां व्युत्क्रमेण च॥६॥
उर्वोरुपरि विप्रेन्द्रे कृत्वा पादतले उभे।
पद्मासनं भवेदेतत्सर्वेषामपि पूजितम्॥७॥
एकं पादमथैकस्मिन्विन्यस्योरुणि संस्थितम्।
इतरस्मिंस्तथा चोरुं वीरासनमुदाहृतम्॥८॥
गुल्फौ च वृषणस्याधः सीवन्याः पार्श्वयोः क्षिपेत्।
दक्षिणं सव्यगुल्फेन दक्षिणेन तथेतरम्॥९॥
हस्तौ च जान्वोः संस्थाप्य स्वाङ्गुलीश्च प्रसार्य च।
व्यात्तवक्त्रो निरीक्षेत नासाग्रं सुसमाहितः॥१०॥
सिंहासनं भवेदेतत्पूजितं योगिभिः सदा।
गुल्फौ च वृष्णस्याधः सीवन्याः पार्श्वयोः क्षिपेत्॥११॥
पार्श्वपादौ च पाणिभ्यां दृढं बुद्ध्वा सुनिश्चलम्।
भद्रासनं भवेदेतत्सर्वव्याधिविषापहम्॥१२॥
संपीडय सीवनीं सूक्ष्मां गुल्फेनैव तु सव्यतः।
सव्यं दक्षिणगुल्फेन मुक्तासनमितीरितम्॥१३॥
मेढ्रादुपरि निक्षिप्य सव्यं गुल्फं तथोपरि।
गुल्फान्तरं च निक्षिप्य मुक्तासनमिदं तु वा॥१४॥
अवष्टभ्य धरां सम्यक् तलाभ्यां तु करद्वयोः।
हस्तयोः कूर्परौ चापि स्थापयन्नाभिपार्श्वयोः॥१५॥

समुन्नतशिरःपादो दण्डवद्व्योम्नि संस्थितः।

मयूरासनमेतत्तु सर्वपापप्रणाशनम्॥ १६॥

सर्वे चाभ्यन्तरा रोगा विनश्यन्ति विषाणि च।

यमैश्च नियमैश्चैव आसनैश्च सुसंयुता॥ १७॥

नाडीशुद्धिं च कृत्वा तु प्राणायामं ततः कुरु॥ १८॥

इति श्रीयोगयाज्ञवल्क्ये तृतीयोऽध्यायः।

चतुर्थोऽध्यायः

श्रुत्वैतद्भाषितं वाक्यं याज्ञवल्क्यस्य धीमतः।

पुनः प्राह महाभागा सभामध्ये तपस्वनी॥ १॥

गार्ग्युवाच--

भगवन्ब्रूहि मे स्वामिन्नाडीशुद्धिं विधानतः।

केनोपायेन शुद्धाः स्युर्नाडयः सर्वदेहिनाम्॥ २॥

उत्पत्तिं चापि नाडीनां चारणं च यथाविधि।

कन्दं च कीदृशं प्रोक्तं कति तिष्ठन्ति वायवः॥ ३॥

स्थानानि चैव वायूनां कर्माणि च पृथक्पृथक्।

विज्ञातव्यानि यान्यस्मिन्देहे देहभृतां वर॥ ४॥

वक्तुमर्हसि तत्सर्वं त्वत्तो वेत्ता न विद्यते।

इत्युक्तो भार्यया तत्र सम्यक् तद्गतमानसः॥ ५॥

गार्गीं तां सुसमालोक्य तत्सर्वं समभाषत।

याज्ञवल्क्य उवाच--

शरीरं तावदेवं हि षण्णवत्यङ्गुलात्मकम्॥ ६॥

विध्येतत्सर्वजन्तूनां स्वाङ्गुलीभिरिति प्रिये।

शरीरादधिकः प्राणो द्वादशाङ्गुलमानतः॥७॥

चतुर्दशाङ्गुलं केचिद्वदन्ति मुनिसत्तमाः।

द्वादशाङ्गुल एवेति वदन्ति ज्ञानिनो नराः॥८॥

आत्मस्थमनिलं विद्वानात्मस्थेनैव वह्निना।

योगाभ्यासेन यः कुर्यात्समं वा न्यूनमेव वा॥९॥

स एव ब्रह्मविच्छ्रेष्ठः स सम्पूज्यो नरोत्तमः।

आत्मस्थवह्निनैव त्वं योगजेन द्विजोत्तमे॥१०॥

आत्मस्थं मातरिश्वानं योगाभ्यासेन निर्जय।

देहमध्ये शिखिस्थानं तप्तजाम्बूनदप्रभम्॥११॥

त्रिकोणं मनुजानां च चतुरस्रं चतुष्पदाम्।

मण्डलं तत्पतङ्गानां सत्यमेतद्ब्रवीमि ते॥१२॥

तन्मध्ये तु शिखा तन्वी सदा तिष्ठति पावकी।

देहमध्यं च कुत्रेति श्रोतुमिच्छसि चेच्छृणु॥१३॥

गुदात्तु द्व्यङ्गुलादूर्ध्वमधो मेढ्राच्च द्व्यङ्गुलात्।

देहमध्यं तयोर्मध्यं मनुष्याणामितीरितम्॥१४॥

चतुष्पदां तु हृन्मध्यं तिरश्चां तुन्दमध्यमम्।

द्विजानां तु वरारोहे तुन्दमध्यमितीरितम्॥१५॥

कन्दस्थानां मनुष्याणां देहमध्यान्नवाङ्गुलम्।

चतुरङ्गुलमुत्सेधमायामश्च तथाविधः॥१६॥

अण्डाकृतिवदाकारं भूषितं तत्त्वगादिभिः।

चतुष्पदां तिरश्चां च द्विजानां तुन्दमध्यमे॥१७॥

तन्मध्यं नाभिरित्युक्तं नाभौ चक्रसमुद्भवः।

द्वादशारयुतं तच्च तेन देहः प्रतिष्ठितः॥ १८॥

चक्रेऽस्मिन्भ्रमते जीवः पापपुण्यप्रचोदितः।

तन्तुपञ्जरमध्यस्था यथा भ्रमति लूतिका॥ १९॥

जीवस्य मूलचक्रेऽस्मिन्नधः प्राणश्चरत्यसौ।

प्राणारूढो भवेज्जीवः सर्वभूतेषु सर्वदा॥ २०॥

तस्योर्ध्वं कुण्डलीस्थानं नाभेस्तिर्यगथोर्ध्वतः।

अष्टप्रकृतिरूपा सा अष्टधा कुण्डलीकृता॥ २१॥

यथावद्वायुसञ्चारं जलान्नादीनि नित्यशः।

परितः कन्दपार्श्वेषु निरुध्यैव सदा स्थिता॥ २२॥

मुखेनैव समावेष्ट्य ब्रह्मरन्ध्रमुखं तथा।

योगकाले त्वपानेन प्रबोधं याति साग्निना॥ २३॥

स्फुरन्ती हृदयाकाशे नागरूपा महोज्ज्वला।

वायुर्वायुसखेनैव ततो याति सुषुम्णया॥ २४॥

कन्दमध्ये स्थिता नाडी सुषुम्णेति प्रकीर्तिता।

तिष्ठन्ति परितः सर्वाश्चक्रेऽस्मिन्नाडीसंज्ञकाः॥ २५॥

नाडीनामपि सर्वासां मुख्यास्त्वेताश्चतुर्दश।

इडा च पिङ्गला चैव सुषुम्णा च सरस्वती॥ २६॥

वारुणी चैव पूषा च हस्तिजिह्वा यशस्विनी।

विश्वोदरा कुहूश्चैव शङ्खिनी च पयस्विनी॥ २७॥

अलम्बुषा च गान्धारी मुख्याश्चैताश्चतुर्दश।

आसां मुख्यतमास्तिस्रस्तिसृष्वेकोत्तमोत्तमा॥ २८॥

मुक्तिमार्गेति सा प्रोक्ता सुषुम्णा विश्वधारिणी।

कन्दस्य मध्यमे गार्गि सुषुम्णा सुप्रतिष्ठिता॥ २९॥

पृष्ठमध्ये स्थिता नाडी सा हि मूर्ध्नि व्यवस्थिता।

मुक्तिमार्गः सुषुम्णा सा ब्रह्मरन्ध्रेति कीर्तिता॥ ३०॥

अव्यक्ता सैव विज्ञेया सूक्ष्मा सा वैष्णवी स्मृता।

इडा च पिङ्गला चैव तस्याः सव्ये च दक्षिणे॥ ३१॥

इडा तस्याः स्थिता सव्ये दक्षिणे पिङ्गला स्थिता।

इडायां पिङ्गलायां च चरतश्चन्द्रभास्करौ॥ ३२॥

इडायां चन्द्रमा ज्ञेयः पिङ्गलायां रविः स्मृतः।

चन्द्रस्तामस इत्युक्तः सूर्यो राजस उच्यते॥ ३३॥

विषभागो रवेर्भागः सोमभागोऽमृतं स्मृतम्।

तावेव धत्तः सकलं कालं रात्रिदिवात्मकम्॥ ३४॥

भोक्त्री सुषुम्णा कालस्य गुह्यमेतदुदाहृतम्।

सरस्वती कुहुश्चैव सुषुम्णापार्श्वयोः स्थिते॥ ३५॥

गान्धारी हस्तिजिह्वा च इडायाः पृष्ठपार्श्वयोः।

कुहोश्च हस्तिजिह्वाया मध्ये विश्वोदरा स्थिता॥ ३६॥

यशस्विन्याः कुहोर्मध्ये वारुणी च प्रतिष्ठिता।

पूषायाश्च सरस्वत्याः स्थिता मध्ये पयस्विनी॥ ३७॥

गान्धार्याश्च सरस्वत्याः स्थिता मध्ये च शङ्खिनी।

अलम्बुषा च विप्रेन्द्रे कन्दमध्यादधः स्थिता॥ ३८॥

पूर्वभागे सुषुम्णाया आमेढ्रान्ते कुहूः स्थिता।

अधश्चोर्ध्वं च कुण्डल्या वारुणी सर्वगामिनी॥ ३९॥

यशस्विनी च याम्यस्था पादाङ्गुष्ठान्तमिष्यते।

पिङ्गला चोर्ध्वगा याम्ये नासान्तं विद्धि मे प्रिये॥ ४०॥

याम्ये पूषा च नेत्रान्तं पिङ्गलायास्तु पृष्ठतः।

पयस्विनी तथा गार्गि याम्यकर्णान्तिमिष्यते॥ ४१॥

सरस्वती तथा चोर्ध्वमाजिह्वायाः प्रतिष्ठिता।

आसव्यकर्णाद्विप्रेन्द्रे शङ्खिनी चोर्ध्वगा मता॥ ४२॥

गान्धारी सव्यनेत्रान्तमिडायाः पृष्ठतः स्थिता।

इडा च सव्यनासान्तं सव्यभागे व्यवस्थिता॥ ४३॥

हस्तिजिह्वा तथा सव्यपादाङ्गुष्ठान्तमिष्यते।

विश्वोदरा तु या नाडी तुन्दमध्ये व्यवस्थिता॥ ४४॥

अलम्बुषा महाभागे पायुमूलादधोगता।

एतास्त्वन्याः समुत्पन्नाः शिराश्चान्याश्च तास्वपि॥ ४५॥

यथाश्वत्थदले तद्वदब्जपत्रेषु वा शिराः।

नाडीष्वेतासु सर्वासु विज्ञातव्यास्तपोधने॥ ४६॥

प्राणोऽपानःसमानश्च उदानो व्यान एव च।

नागः कूर्मोऽथ कृकरो देवदत्तो धनञ्जयः॥ ४७॥

एते नाडीषु सर्वासु चरन्ति दश वायवः।

एतेषु वायवः पञ्च मुख्याः प्राणादयः स्मृताः॥ ४८॥

तेषु मुख्यतमावेतौ प्राणापानौ नरोत्तमे।

प्राण एवतयोर्मुख्यः सर्वप्राणभृतां सदा॥ ४९॥

आस्यनासिकयोर्मध्ये हृन्मध्ये नाभिमध्यमे।

प्राणालय इति प्राहुः पादाङ्गुष्ठेऽपि केचन॥ ५०॥

अधश्चोर्ध्वं च कुण्डल्याः परीतः प्राणसंज्ञकः।

तिष्ठन्नेतेषु सर्वेषु प्रकाशयति दीपवत्॥५१॥

अपाननिलयं केचिद् गुदमेढ्रोरुजानुषु।

उदरे वृषणे कट्यां जङ्घे नाभौ वदन्ति हि॥५२॥

गुदाग्न्यागारयोस्तिष्ठन्मध्येऽपानः प्रभञ्जनः।

अधश्चोर्ध्वं च कुण्डल्याः प्रकाशयति दीपवत्॥५३॥

व्यानः श्रोत्राक्षिमध्ये च कृकट्यां गुल्फयोरपि।

घ्राणे गले स्फिजोर्देशे तिष्ठत्यत्र न संशयः॥५४॥

उदानः सर्वसन्धिस्थः पादयोर्हस्तयोरपि।

समानः सर्वगात्रेषु सर्व व्याप्य व्यवस्थितः॥५५॥

भुक्तं सर्वरसं गात्रे व्यापयन्वह्निना सह।

द्विसप्ततिसहस्रेषु नाडीमर्गेषु सञ्चरेत्॥५६॥

समानवायुरेवैकः साग्निर्व्याप्य व्यवस्थितः।

अग्निभिः सह सर्वत्र साङ्गोपाङ्गकलेवरे॥५७॥

नागादि वायवः पञ्च त्वगस्थ्यादिषु संस्थिताः।

तुन्दस्थं जलमन्नं च रसानि च समीकृतम्॥५८॥

तुन्दमध्यगतः प्राणस्तानि कुर्यात्पृथक्पृथक्।

पुनरग्नौ जलं स्थाप्य त्वन्नादीनि जलोपरि॥५९॥

स्वयं ह्यपानं संप्राप्य तेनैव सह मारुतः।

प्रवाति ज्वलनं तत्र देहमध्यगतं पुनः॥६०॥

वायुना वातितो वह्निरपानेन शनैः शनैः।

तदा ज्वलति विप्रेन्द्रे स्वकुले देहमध्यमे॥६१॥

ज्वालाभिर्ज्वलनस्तत्र प्राणेन प्रेरितस्ततः।

जलमत्युष्णमकरोत्कोष्ठमध्यगतं तदा॥६२॥

अन्नं व्यञ्जनसंयुक्तं जलोपरि समर्पितम्।

ततः सुपक्वमकरोद्वह्निः सन्तप्तवारिणा॥६३॥

स्वेदमूत्रे जलं स्यातां वीर्यरूपं रसो भवेत्।

पूरीषमन्नं स्याद्गार्गि प्राणः कुर्यात्पृथक्पृथक्॥६४॥

समानवायुना सार्धं रसं सर्वासु नाडीषु।

व्यापयञ्छ्वासरूपेण देहे चरति मारुतः॥६५॥

व्योमरन्ध्रैश्च नवभिः विण्मूत्रादिविसर्जनम्।

कुर्वन्ति वायवः सर्वे शरीरेषु निरन्तरम्॥६६॥

निःश्वासोच्छ्वासकासाश्च प्राणकर्मेति कीर्त्यते।

अपानवायोः कर्मैतद्विण्मूत्रादिविसर्जनम्॥६७॥

हानोपादानचेष्टादि व्यानकर्मेति चेष्यते।

उदानकर्म तत्प्रोक्तं देहस्योन्नयनादि यत्॥६८॥

पोषणादि समानस्य शरीरे कर्म कीर्तितम्।

उद्गारादि गुणो यस्तु नागकर्मेति कीर्त्यते॥६९॥

निमीलनादि कूर्मस्य क्षुतं वै कृकरस्य च।

देवदत्तस्य विप्रेन्द्रे तन्द्रीकर्मेति कीर्तितम्॥७०॥

धनञ्जयस्य शोफादि सर्वं कर्म प्रकीर्तितम्।

ज्ञात्वैवं नाडीसंस्थानं वायूनां स्थानकर्मणी॥७१॥

विधिनोक्तेन मार्गेण नाडीसंशोधनं कुरु॥७२॥

इति श्री योगयाज्ञवल्क्ये चतुर्थोऽध्यायः।

पञ्चमोऽध्यायः

गार्ग्युवाच--

भगवन्ब्रह्मविच्छ्रेष्ठ सर्वशास्त्रविशारद।

केनोपयेन शुद्धाः स्युर्नाडयो मे त्वं वद प्रभो॥ १॥

इत्युक्तो ब्रह्मवादिन्या ब्रह्मविद्ब्राह्मणस्तदा।

तं समालोक्य कृपया नाडीशुद्धिमभाषत॥ २॥

याज्ञवल्क्य उवाच--

विध्युक्तकर्मसंयुक्तः कामसङ्कल्पवर्जितः।

यमैश्च नियमैर्युक्तः सर्वसङ्गविवर्जितः॥ ३॥

कृतविद्यो जितक्रोधः सत्यधर्मपरायणः।

गुरुशुश्रुषणरतः पितृमातृपरायणः॥ ४॥

स्वाश्रमस्थः सदाचारः विद्वद्भिश्च सुशिक्षितः।

तपोवनं सुसम्प्राप्य फलमूलोदकान्वितम्॥ ५॥

तत्र रम्ये शुचौ देशे ब्रह्मघोषसमन्विते।

स्वधर्मनिरतैः शान्तैर्ब्रह्मविद्भिः समावृते॥ ६॥

वारिभिश्च सुसम्पूर्णे पुष्पैर्नानाविधैर्युते।

फलमूलैश्च सम्पूर्णे सर्वकामफलप्रदे॥ ७॥

देवालये वा नद्यां वा ग्रामे वा नगरेऽथवा।

सुशोभनं मठं कृत्वा सर्वरक्षासमन्वितम्॥ ८॥

त्रिकालस्नानसंयुक्तः स्वधर्मनिरतः सदा।

वेदान्तश्रवणं कुर्वंस्तस्मिन्योगं समभ्यसेत्॥ ९॥

केचिद्वदन्ति मुनयस्तपःस्वाध्यायसंयुताः।

स्वधर्मनिरताः शान्तास्तन्त्रेषु च सदा रताः॥ १०॥

निर्जने निलये रम्ये वातातपविवर्जिते।
विध्युक्तकर्मसंयुक्तः शुचिर्भूत्वा समाहितः॥ ११॥
मन्त्रैर्न्यस्ततनुर्धीरः सितभस्मधरः सदा।
मृद्वासनोपरि कुशान्समास्तीर्य ततोऽजिनम्॥ १२॥
विनायकं सुसम्पूज्य फलमूलोदकादिभिः।
इष्टदेवं गुरुं नत्वा तत आरुह्य चासनम्॥ १३॥
प्राङ्मुखोदङ्मुखो वापि जितासनगतः स्वयम्।
समग्रीवशिरःकायः संवृतास्यः सुनिश्चलः॥ १४॥
नासाग्रदृक् सदा सम्यक् सव्ये न्यस्येतरं करम्।
नासाग्रे शशभृद्बिम्बं ज्योत्स्नाजालवितानितम्॥ १५॥
सप्तमस्य तु वर्गस्य चतुर्थं बिन्दुसंयुतम्।
स्रवन्तममृतं पश्यन्नेत्राभ्यां सुसमाहितः॥ १६॥
इडया वायुमारोप्य पूरयित्वोदरस्थितम्।
ततोऽग्निं देहमध्यस्थं ध्यायन्ज्वालावलीयुतम्॥ १७॥
रेफं च बिन्दुसंयुक्तमग्निमण्डलसंस्थितम्।
ध्यायन्विरेचयेत्पश्चान्मन्दं पिङ्गलया पुनः॥ १८॥
पुनः पिङ्गलयापूर्य प्राणं दक्षिणतः सुधीः।
पुनर्विरेचयेद्धीमानिडया तु शनैः शनैः॥ १९॥
त्रिचतुर्वत्सरं वाथ त्रिचतुर्मासमेव वा।
षट्कृत्व आचरेन्नित्यं रहस्येवं त्रिसन्धिषु॥ २०॥
नाडीशुद्धिमवाप्नोति पृथक् चिह्नोपलक्षिताम्।
शरीरलघुता दीप्तिर्वह्नेर्जठरवर्तिनः॥ २१॥

नादाभिव्यक्तिरित्येते चिह्नं तत्सिद्धिसूचकम्।

यावदेतानि सम्पश्येत्तावदेव समाचरेत्॥ २२॥

इति श्रीयोगयाज्ञवल्क्ये पञ्चमोऽध्यायः।

षष्ठोऽध्यायः

याज्ञवल्क्य उवाच--

प्राणायाममथादीनां प्रवक्ष्यामि विधानतः।

समाहितमनास्त्वं च शृणु गार्गि वरानने॥ १॥

प्राणापानसमायोगः प्राणायाम इतीरितः।

प्राणायाम इति प्रोक्तो रेचकपूरककुम्भकैः॥ २॥

वर्णत्रयात्मका ह्येते रेचकपूरककुम्भकाः।

स एष प्रणवः प्रोक्तः प्राणायामश्च तन्मयः॥ ३॥

इडया वायुमारोप्य पूरयित्वोदरस्थितम्।

शनैः षोडशभिर्मात्रैरकारं तत्र संस्मरेत्॥ ४॥

धारयेत् पूरितं पश्चाच्चतुःषष्ठ्या तु मात्रया।

उकारमूर्तिमत्रापि संस्मरन्प्रणवं जपेत्॥ ५॥

यावद्वा शक्यते तावद्धारणं जपसंयुतम्।

पूरितं रेचयेत् पश्चात्प्राणं बाह्यानिलान्वितम्॥ ६॥

शनैः पिङ्गलया गार्गि द्वात्रिंशन्मात्रया पुनः।

मकारमूर्तिमत्रापि संस्मरन्प्रणवं जपेत्॥ ७॥

प्राणायामो भवेदेषः पुनश्चैवं समभ्यसेत्।

ततः पिङ्गलयापूर्य मात्रैः षोडशभिस्तथा॥ ८॥

उकारमूर्तिमत्रापि संस्मरन्सुसमाहितः।

पूरितं धारयेत्प्राणं प्रणवं विंशतिद्वयम्॥ ९॥

जपेदत्र स्मरन्मूर्तिं मकाराख्यं महेश्वरम्।

यावद्वा शक्यते पश्चाद्रेचयेदिडयानिलम्॥ १०॥

एवमेव पुनः कुर्यादिडयापूर्य पूर्ववत्।

नाड्या प्राणं समारोप्य पूरयित्वोदरस्थितम्॥ ११॥

प्रणवेन सुसंयुक्तां व्याहृतीभिश्च संयुताम्।

गायत्रीं च जपेद्विप्रः प्राणसम्यमने त्रयः॥ १२॥

पुनश्चैवं त्रिभिः कुर्यात्पुनश्चैव त्रिसन्धिषु।

यद्वा समभ्यसेन्नित्यं वैदिकं लौकिकं तु वा॥ १३॥

प्राणसंयमने विद्वान्जपेत्तद्विंशतिद्वयम्।

ब्राह्मणः श्रुतसम्पन्नः स्वधर्मनिरतः सदा॥ १४॥

स वैदिकं जपेन्मन्त्रं लौकिकं न कदाचन।

केचिद्भूतहितार्थाय जपमिच्छन्ति लौकिकम्॥ १५॥

द्विजवत्क्षात्रस्योक्तः प्राणसंयमने जपः।

वैश्यानां धर्मयुक्तानां स्त्रीशूद्राणां तपस्विनाम्॥ १६॥

प्राणसंयमने गार्गि मन्त्रं प्रणववर्जितम्।

नमोन्तं शिवमन्त्रं वा वैष्णवं वेष्यते बुधैः॥ १७॥

यद्वा समभ्यसेच्छूद्रो लौकिकं विधिपूर्वकम्।

प्राणसंयमने स्त्री च जपेत्तद्विंशतिद्वयम्॥ १८॥

न वैदिकं जपेच्छूद्रः स्त्रियश्च न कदाचन।

स्वाश्रमस्थस्य वैश्यस्य केचिदिच्छन्ति वैदिकम्॥ १९॥

सन्ध्ययोरुभयोर्नित्यं गायत्र्या प्रणवेन वा।

प्राणसंयमनं कुर्यात् ब्राह्मणो वेदपारगः ॥ २० ॥

नित्यमेव प्रकुर्वीत प्राणायामांस्तु षोडश।

अपि भ्रूणहनं मासात्पुनन्त्यहरहः कृताः ॥ २१ ॥

ऋतुत्रयात्पुनन्त्येनं जन्मान्तरकृतादघात्।

वत्सराद्ब्रह्महा शुद्ध्येत्तस्मान्नित्यं समभ्यसेत् ॥ २२ ॥

योगाभ्यासरतास्त्वेवं स्वधर्मनिरताश्च ये।

प्राणसंयमनेनैव सर्वे मुक्ता भवन्ति हि ॥ २३ ॥

बाह्यादापूरणं वायोरुदरे पूरको हि सः।

सम्पूर्णकुम्भवद्वायोर्धारणं कुम्भको भवेत् ॥ २४ ॥

बहिर्यद्रेचनं वायोरुदराद्रेचकः स्मृतः।

प्रस्वेदजनको यस्तु प्राणायामेषु सोऽधमः ॥ २५ ॥

कम्पको मध्यमः प्रोक्त उत्थानश्चोत्तमो भवेत्।

पूर्वं पूर्वं प्रकुर्वीत यावदुत्तमसम्भवः ॥ २६ ॥

सम्भवत्युत्तमे गार्गि प्राणायामे सुखी भवेत्।

प्राणो लयति तेनैव देहस्यान्तस्ततोऽधिकः ॥ २७ ॥

देहश्चोत्तिष्ठते तेन कृतासनपरिग्रहः।

निःश्वासोच्छ्वासकौ तस्य न विद्येते कथंचन ॥ २८ ॥

देहे यद्यपि तौ स्यातां स्वाभाविकगुणावुभौ।

तथापि नश्यतस्तेन प्राणायामोत्तमेन हि ॥ २९ ॥

तयोर्नाशे समर्थः स्यात्कर्तुं केवलकुम्भकम्।

रेचकं पूरकं मुक्त्वा सुखं यद्वायुधारणम् ॥ ३० ॥

प्राणायामोऽयमित्युक्तः स वै केवलकुम्भकः।

रेच्य चापूर्य यः कुर्यात्स वै सहितकुम्भकः ॥ ३१ ॥

सहितं केवलं चाथ कुम्भकं नित्यमभ्यसेत्।

यावत्केवलसिद्धिः स्यात्तावत्सहितमभ्यसेत्॥ ३२ ॥

केवले कुम्भके सिद्धे रेचपूरणवर्जिते।

न तस्य दुर्लभं किञ्चित्त्रिषु लोकेषु विद्यते॥ ३३ ॥

मनोजवत्वं लभते पलितादि च नश्यति।

मुक्तेरयं महामार्गो मकाराख्यान्तरात्मनः॥ ३४॥

नादं चोत्पादयत्येषः कुम्भकः प्राणसंयमः।

प्राणसंसयनं नाम देहे प्राणस्य धारणम्॥ ३५॥

एषः प्राणजयोपायः सर्वमृत्यूपघातकः।

किंचित्प्राणजयोपायं तव वक्ष्यामि तत्त्वतः॥ ३६ ॥

बाह्यात्प्राणं समाकृष्य पूरयित्वोदरस्थितम्।

नाभिमध्ये च नासाग्रे पादाङ्गुष्ठे च यत्नतः॥ ३७॥

धारयेन्मनसा प्राणं सन्ध्याकालेषु सर्वदा।

सर्वरोगविनिर्मुक्तो जीवेद्योगी गतक्लमः॥ ३८॥

नासाग्रे धारणं गार्गि वायोर्विजयकारणम्।

सर्वरोगविनाशः स्यान्नाभिमध्ये च धारणात्॥ ३९॥

शरीर लघुतां याति पादाङ्गुष्ठे च धारणात्।

रसनावायुमाकृष्य यः पिबेत्सततं नरः॥४०॥

श्रमदाहौ न तस्यास्तां नश्यन्ति व्याधयस्तथा।

सन्ध्ययोब्राह्मकाले वा वायुमकृष्य यः पिबेत्॥ ४१ ॥

त्रिमासात्तस्य कल्याणि जायते वाक्सरस्वती।

षण्मासाभ्यासयोगेन महारोगैः प्रमुच्यते॥ ४२॥

आत्मन्यात्मानमारोप्य कुण्डल्यां यस्तु धारयेत्।

क्षयरोगादयस्तस्य नश्यन्तीत्यपरे विदुः॥ ४३॥

जिह्वया वायुमानीय जिह्वामूले निरोधयन्।

यः पिबेदमृतं विद्वान्सकलं भद्रमश्नुते॥ ४४॥

आत्मन्यात्मानमिडया समानीय भ्रुवोन्तरे।

पिबेद्यस्त्रिदशाहारं व्याधिभिः स विमुच्यते॥ ४५॥

नाडीभ्यां वायुमारोप्य नाभौ वा तुन्दपार्श्वयोः।

घटिकैकां वहेद्यस्तु व्याधिभिः सोऽभिमुच्यते॥ ४६॥

मासमेकं त्रिसन्ध्यायां जिह्वयारोप्य मारुतम्।

पिबेद्यस्त्रिदशाहारं धारयेत्तुन्दमध्यमे॥ ४७॥

गुल्माष्ठीला प्लीहा चान्ये त्रिदोषजनितास्तथा।

तुन्दमध्यगता रोगाः सर्वे नश्यन्ति तस्य वै॥ ४८॥

ज्वराः सर्वे विनश्यन्ति विषाणि विविधानि च।

बहुनोक्तेन किं गार्गि पलितादि च नश्यति॥ ४९॥

एवं वायुजयोपायः प्राणस्य तु वरानने।

शक्यमासनमास्थाय समाहितमनास्तथा॥ ५०॥

करणानि वशीकृत्य विषयेभ्यो बलात्सुधीः।

अपानमूर्ध्वमाकृष्य प्रणवेन समाहितः॥ ५१॥

हस्ताभ्यां बन्धयेत्सम्यक्कर्णादि करणानि च।

अङ्गुष्ठाभ्यामुभे श्रोत्रे तर्जनीभ्यां च चक्षुषी॥ ५२॥

नासापुटौ मध्यमाभ्यां प्रच्छाद्य करणानि वै।

आनन्दानुभवं यावत्तावन्मूर्द्धनि धारयेत्॥५३॥

प्राणः प्रयात्यनेनैव ततस्त्वायुर्विघातकृत्।

ब्रह्मरन्ध्रे सुषुम्णायां मृणालान्तरसूत्रवत्॥५४॥

नादोत्पत्तिस्त्वनेनैव शुद्धस्फटिकसन्निभा।

आमूर्ध्नो वर्तते नादो वीणादण्डवदुत्थितः॥५५॥

शंखध्वनिनिभस्त्वादौ मध्ये मेघध्वनिर्यथा।

व्योमरन्ध्रे गते नादे गिरिप्रस्रवणं यथा॥५६॥

व्योमरन्ध्रे गते वायौ चित्ते चात्मनि संस्थिते।

तदानन्दी भवेद्देही वायुस्तेन जितो भवेत्॥५७॥

योगिनस्त्वपरे ह्यत्र वदन्ति समचेतसः।

प्राणायामपराः पूता रेचपूरणवर्जिताः॥५८॥

दक्षिणेतरगुल्फेन सीवनीं पीडयेत् शिराम्।

अधस्तादण्डयोः सूक्ष्मां सव्योपरि च दक्षिणम्॥५९॥

जङ्घोर्वोरन्तरं गार्गि निश्छिद्रं बन्धयेद्दृढम्।

समग्रीवशिरस्कन्धः समपृष्ठः समोदरः॥६०॥

नेत्राभ्यां दक्षिणं गुल्फं लोकयन्नुपरिस्थितम्।

धारयन्मनसा सार्धं व्याहरन्प्रणवाक्षरम्॥६१॥

आसने नान्यधीरास्ते द्विजो रहसि नित्यशः।

क्षत्रियश्च वरारोहे व्याहरन्प्रणवाक्षरम्॥६२॥

आसने नान्यधीरस्ते रहस्येव जितेन्द्रियः।

वैश्याः शूद्राः स्त्रियश्चान्ये योगाभ्यासरताः नराः॥६३॥

शैवं वा वैष्णवं वाथ व्याहरन्नन्यमेव वा।

आसने नान्यधीरस्ते दीपं हस्ते विलोकयन्॥ ६४॥

आयुर्विघातकृत्प्राणस्त्वनेनाग्निकुलं गतः।

धूमध्वजजयं यावन्नान्यधीरेवमभ्यसेत्॥ ६५॥

धारणं कुर्वतस्तस्य शक्तिः स्यादिष्टभोजने।

देहश्च लघुतां याति जठराग्निश्च वर्धते॥ ६६॥

दृष्टचिह्नस्ततस्तस्मान्मनसारोप्य मारुतम्।

मन्त्रमुच्चारयन्दीर्घं नाभिमध्ये निरोधयेत्॥ ६७॥

यावन्मनो लयत्यस्मिन्नाभौ सवितृमण्डले।

तावत्समभ्यसेद्विद्वान्नियतो नियतासनः॥ ६८॥

एतेन नाभिमध्यस्थधारणेनैव मारुतः।

कुण्डलीं याति वह्निश्च दहत्यत्र न संशयः॥ ६९॥

सन्तप्ता वह्निना तत्र वायुना चालिता स्वयम्।

प्रसार्य फणभृद्भोगं प्रबोधं याति सा तदा॥ ७०॥

प्रबुद्धे संसरत्यस्मिन्नाभिमूले तु चक्रिणि।

ब्रह्मरन्ध्रे सुषुम्णायां प्रयाति प्राणसंज्ञकः॥ ७१॥

संप्राप्ते मारुते तस्मिन्सुषुम्णायां वरानने।

मन्त्रमुच्चार्य मनसा हृन्मध्ये धारयेत्पुनः॥ ७२॥

हृदयात्कण्ठकूपे च भ्रुवोर्मध्ये च धारयेत्।

तस्मादारोप्य मनसा साग्निं प्राणमनन्यधीः॥ ७३॥

धारयेद्व्योम्नि विप्रेन्द्रे व्याहरन्प्रणवाक्षरम्।

वायुना पूरिते व्योम्नि साङ्गोपाङ्गे कलेवरे॥ ७४॥

तदात्मा राजते तत्र यथा व्योम्नि विकर्तनः।

शरीरं विसुसृक्षुश्चेदेवं सम्यक् समाचरन्॥ ७५॥
एकाक्षरं परं ब्रह्म ध्यायन्प्रणवमीश्वरम्।
संभिद्य मनसा मूर्ध्नि ब्रह्मरन्ध्रं सवायुना॥ ७६॥
प्राणमुन्मोचयेत्पश्चान्महाप्राणे खमध्यमे।
देहातीते जगत्प्राणे शून्ये नित्ये ध्रुवे पदे॥ ७७॥
आकाशे परमानन्दे स्वात्मानं योजयेद्धिया।
ब्रह्मेवासौ भवेद्गार्गि न पुनर्जन्मभाग्भवेत्॥ ७८॥
तस्मात्त्वं च वरारोहे नित्यं कर्म समाचार।
सन्ध्याकालेषु वा नित्यं प्राणसंयमनं कुरु॥ ७९॥
प्राणायामपराः सर्वे प्राणायामपरायणाः।
प्राणायामविशुद्धा ये ते यान्ति परमां गतिम्॥ ८०॥
प्राणायामादृते नान्यत्तारकं नरकादपि।
संसारार्णवमग्नानां तारकः प्राणसंयमः॥ ८१॥
तस्मात्त्वं विधिमार्गेण नित्यं कर्म समाचर।
विधिनोक्तेन मार्गेण प्राणसंयमनं कुरु॥ ८२॥
इति श्रीयोगयाज्ञवल्क्ये षष्ठोऽध्यायः॥
नासाग्रे दृक् सदा सम्यक् सव्ये न्यस्येतरं करम्।
नासाग्रे शशभृद्बिम्बे ज्योत्सनाजालवितानके॥ १॥
अम्बोमा सहितं शुभ्रं सोमसूर्याग्निलोचनम्।
पञ्चवक्त्रं महादेवं चन्द्रशेखरमीखरम्॥ २॥
नन्दिवाहनसंयुक्तं सर्वदेवसमन्वितम्।
प्रसन्नं सर्ववरदं ध्यायेत्सर्वायुधं शिवम्॥ ३॥

यो वेदादौ स्वरः प्रोक्तो वेदान्ते च प्रतिष्ठितः।

अकारमूर्तिरेतेषां रक्ताङ्गी हंसवाहिनी॥४॥

दण्डहस्ता सती बाला गायत्रीत्यवधार्यताम्।

उकारमूर्तिरेतेषां कृष्णाङ्गी वृषवाहनी॥५॥

चक्रहस्ता सती चैव सावित्रीत्यवधार्यताम्।

मकारमूर्तिरेतेषां श्वेताङ्गी तार्क्ष्यवाहिनी॥६॥

शूलानन्दमयी वृद्धा सरस्वत्यवधार्यताम्।

माहेश्वरीति सा प्राज्ञैः पश्चिमा परिकीर्तिता॥७॥

सृष्टिस्थित्यन्तकालाद्या मकारोऽप्यन्तकात्मकः।

अक्षरत्रयमेवैतत्कारणत्रयमिष्यते॥८॥

त्रयाणां कारणं ब्रह्म सद्रूपं सर्वकारणम्।

एकाक्षरं परं ज्योतिस्तमाहुः प्रणवं बुधाः॥९॥

एवं ज्ञात्वा विधानेन प्रणवेन समन्वितम्।

प्राणायामं ततः कुर्याद्रेचपूरककुम्भकैः॥१०॥

सप्तमोऽध्यायः

याज्ञवल्क्य उवाच--

उक्तान्येतानि चत्वारि योगाङ्गानि द्विजोत्तमे।

प्रत्याहारादि चत्वारि श्रृणुष्वाभ्यन्तराणि च॥१॥

इन्द्रियाणां विचरतां विषयेषु स्वभावतः।

बलादाहरणं तेषां प्रत्याहारः स उच्यते॥२॥

यद्यत्पश्यसि तत्सर्वं पश्येदात्मवदात्मनि।

प्रत्याहारः स च प्रोक्तो योगविद्भिर्महात्मभिः॥३॥

कर्माणि यानि नित्यानि विहितानि शरीरिणाम्।

तेषामात्मन्यनुष्ठानं मनसा यद्बहिर्विना॥४॥

प्रत्याहारो भवेत्सोऽपि योगसाधनमुत्तमम्।

प्रत्याहारः प्रशस्तोऽयं सेवितो योगिभिः सदा॥५॥

अष्टादशसु यद्वायोर्मर्मस्थानेषु धारणम्।

स्थानात्स्थानात्समाकृष्य प्रत्याहारो निगद्यते॥६॥

अश्विनौ च तथा ब्रूतां गार्गि देवभिषग्वरौ।

मर्मस्थानानि सिद्ध्यर्थं शरीरे योगमोक्षयोः॥७॥

तानि सर्वाणि वक्ष्यामि यथावच्छृणु सुव्रते।

पादाङ्गुष्ठौ च गुल्फौ च जङ्घामध्ये तथैव च॥८॥

चित्योर्मूलं च जान्वोश्च मध्ये चोरुद्वयस्य च।

पायुमूलं ततः पश्चाद्देहमध्यं च मेढ्रकम्॥९॥

नाभिश्च हृदयं गार्गि कण्ठकूपस्तथैव च।

तालुमूलं च नासाया मूलं चाक्ष्णोश्च मण्डले॥१०॥

भ्रुवोर्मध्यं ललाटं च मूर्धा च मुनिसत्तमे।

मर्मस्थानानि चैतानि मानं तेषां पृथक् श्रृणु॥११॥

पादान्मानं तु गुल्फस्य सार्धाङ्गुलचतुष्टयम्।

गुल्फाज्जङ्घस्य मध्यं तु विज्ञेयं तद्दशाङ्गुलम्॥१२॥

जङ्घमध्याच्चित्योर्मूलं यत्तदेकादशाङ्गुलम्।

चित्योर्मूलाद्वरारोहे जानुः स्यादङ्गुलिद्वयम्॥१३॥

जान्वोर्नवाङ्गुलं प्राहुरूरुमध्यं मुनीश्वराः।

ऊरुमध्यात्तथा गार्गि पायुमूलं नवाङ्गुलम्॥१४॥

देहमध्यं तथा पायोर्मूलादर्धाङ्गुलद्वयम्।

देहमध्यात्तथा मेढ्रं तद्वत्सार्धाङ्गुलद्वयम्॥ १५॥

मेढ्रान्नाभिश्च विज्ञेया गार्गि सार्धदशाङ्गुलम्।

चतुर्दशाङ्गुलं नाभेर्हृन्मध्यं च वरानने॥ १६॥

षडङ्गुलं तु हृन्मध्यात्कण्ठकूपं तथैव च।

कण्ठकूपाच्च जिह्वाया मूलं स्याच्चतुरङ्गुलम्॥ १७॥

नासामूलं तु जिह्वाया मूलाच्च चतुरङ्गुलं।

नेत्रस्थानं तु तन्मूलादर्धाङ्गुलमितीष्यते॥ १८॥

तस्मादर्धाङ्गुलं विद्धि भ्रुवोरन्तरमात्मनः।

ललाटाख्यं भ्रुवोर्मध्यादूर्ध्वं स्यादङ्गुलद्वयम्॥ १९॥

ललाटाद्व्योमसंज्ञं स्यादङ्गुलित्रयमेव हि।

स्थानेष्वेतेषु मनसा वायुमारोप्य धारयेत्॥ २०।

स्थानात्स्थानात्समाकृष्य प्रत्याहारं प्रकुर्वतः।

सर्वे रोगा विनश्यन्ति योगाः सिद्ध्यन्ति तस्य वै॥ २१॥

वदन्ति योगिनः केचिद्योगेषु कुशला नराः।

प्रत्याहारं वरारोहे शृणु त्वं तद्वदाम्यहम्॥ २२॥

सम्पूर्णकुम्भवद्वायुमङ्गुष्ठान्मूर्धमध्यतः।

धारयेदनिलं बुद्ध्या प्राणायामप्रचोदितः॥ २३॥

व्योमरन्ध्रात्समाकृष्य ललाटे धारयेत्पुनः।

ललाटाद्वायुमाकृष्य भ्रुवोर्मध्ये निरोधयेत्॥ २४॥

भ्रुवोर्मध्यात्समाकृष्य नेत्रमध्ये निरोधयेत्।

नेत्रात्प्राणं समाकृष्य नासामूले निरोधयेत्॥ २५॥

नासामूलात्तु जिह्वाया मूले प्राणं निरोधयेत्।
जिह्वामूलात्समाकृष्य कण्ठमूले निरोधयेत्॥ २६ ॥
कण्ठमूलात्तु हृन्मध्ये हृदयन्नाभिमध्यमे।
नाभिमध्यात्पुनर्मेढ्रे मेढ्राद्वह्न्यालये ततः॥ २७॥
देहमध्याद्गुदे गार्गि गुदादेवोरुमूलके।
ऊरुमूलात्तयोर्मध्ये तस्माज्जान्वोर्निरोधयेत्॥ २८॥
चितिमूले ततस्तस्माज्जङ्घयोर्मध्यमे तथा।
जङ्घामध्यात्समाकृष्य वायुं गुल्फे निरोधयेत्॥ २९॥
गुल्फादङ्गुष्ठयोर्गार्गि पादयोस्तन्निरोधयेत्।
स्थानात्स्थानात्समाकृष्य यस्त्वेवम् धारयेत् सुधीः॥ ३०॥
सर्वपापविशुद्धात्मा जीवेदाचन्द्रतारकम्।
एतत्तु योगसिद्ध्यर्थमगस्त्येनापि कीर्तितम्॥ ३१॥
प्रत्याहारेषु सर्वेषु प्रशस्तमिति योगिभिः।
नाडीभ्यां वायुमापूर्य कुण्डल्याः पार्श्वयोः क्षिपेत्॥ ३२॥
धारयेद्युगपत्सोऽपि भवरोगाद्विमुच्यते।
पूर्ववद्वायुमारोप्य हृदयव्योम्नि धारयत्॥ ३३॥
सोऽपि याति वरारोहे परमात्मपदं नरः।
व्याधयः किं पुनस्तस्य बाह्याभ्यन्तरवर्तिनः॥ ३४॥
नासाभ्यां वायुमारोप्य पूरयित्वोदरस्थितम्।
भ्रुवोर्मध्याल्लुशोः पश्चात्समारोप्य समाहितः॥ ३५॥
धारयेत्क्षणमात्रं वा सोऽपि याति परां गतिम्।
किं पुनर्बहुनोक्तेन नित्यं कर्म समाचरन्॥ ३६॥

आत्मनः प्राणमारोप्य भ्रुवोर्मध्ये सुषुम्णया।

यावन्मनो लयत्यस्मिन्स्तावत्संयमनं कुरु॥ ३७॥

इति श्रीयोगयज्ञवल्क्ये सप्त्मोऽध्यायः॥

अष्टमोऽध्यायः

याज्ञवल्क्य उवाच--

अथेदानीं प्रवक्ष्यामि धारणाः पञ्च तत्वतः।

समाहितमनास्त्वं च श्रृणु गार्गि तपोधने॥ १॥

यमादिगुणयुक्तस्य मनसः स्थितिरात्मनि।

धारणेत्युच्यते सद्भिः शास्त्रतात्पर्यवेदिभिः॥ २॥

अस्मिन्ब्रह्मपुरे गार्गि यदिदं हृदयाम्बुजम्।

तस्मिन्नेवान्तराकाशे यद्बाह्याकाशधारणम्॥ ३॥

एषा च धारणेत्युक्ता योगशास्त्रविशारदैः।

तान्त्रिकैर्योगशास्त्रज्ञैर्विद्वद्भिश्च सुशिक्षितैः॥ ४॥

धारणाः पञ्चधा प्रोक्तास्ताश्च सर्वाः पृथक् श्रृणु।

भूमिरापस्तथा तेजो वायुराकाशमेव च॥ ५॥

एतेषु पञ्चदेवानां धारणं पञ्चधोच्यते।

पादादिजानुपर्यन्तं पृथिवीस्थानमुच्यते॥ ६॥

आजानोः पायुपर्यन्तमपां स्थानं प्रकीर्तितम्।

आपायोर्हृदयान्तं यद्वह्निस्थानं तदुच्यते॥ ७॥

आहृन्मध्याद्भ्रुवोर्मध्यं यावद्वायुकुलं स्मृतम्।

आभ्रूमध्यात्तु मूर्धान्तमाकाशमिति चोच्यते॥ ८॥

अत्र केचिद्वदन्त्यन्ये योगपण्डितमानिनः।

आजानोर्नाभिपर्यन्तमपांस्थानमिति द्विजाः ॥ ९ ॥

नाभिमध्याद्गलान्तं यद्वह्निस्थानं तदुच्यते।

आगलात्तु ललाटान्तं वायुस्थानमितीरितं ॥ १० ॥

ललाटाद्रन्ध्रपर्यन्तमाकाशस्थानमुच्यते।

अयुक्तमेतदित्युक्तं शास्त्रतात्पर्यवेदिभिः ॥ ११ ॥

यदि स्याज्ज्वलनस्थानं देहमध्ये वरानने।

अयुक्ता कारणे वह्नौ कार्यरूपस्य संस्थितिः ॥ १२ ॥

कार्यकारणसंयोगे कार्यहानिः कथं भवेत्।

दृष्टं तत्कार्यरूपेषु मृदात्मकघटादिषु ॥ १३ ॥

पृथिव्यां धारयेद्वार्गि ब्रह्माणं परमेष्ठिनम्।

विष्णुमप्स्वनले रुद्रमीश्वरं वायुमण्डले ॥ १४ ॥

सदाशिवं तथा व्योम्नि धारयेत्सुसमाहितः।

पृथिव्यां वायुमास्थाय लकारेण समन्वितम् ॥ १५ ॥

ध्यायंश्चतुर्भुजाकारं ब्रह्माणं सृष्टिकारणम्।

धारयेत्पञ्च घटिकाः पृथिवीजयमाप्नुयात् ॥ १६ ॥

वारुणे वायुमारोप्य वकारेण समन्वितम्।

स्मरन्नारायणं सौम्यं चतुर्बाहुं किरीटिनम् ॥ १७ ॥

शुद्धस्फतिकसङ्काशं पीतवाससमच्युतम्।

धारयेत्पञ्च घटिकाः सर्वरोगैः प्रमुच्यते ॥ १८ ॥

वह्नौ चानिलमारोप्य रेफाक्षरसमन्वितम्।

त्र्यक्षं वरप्रदं रुद्रं तरुणादित्यसन्निभम् ॥ १९ ॥

भस्मोध्दूलितसर्वाङ्गं सुप्रसन्नमनुस्मरन्।

धारयेत्पञ्च घटिकाः वह्निनासौ न दह्यते॥ २०॥

मारुत मारुतस्थाने यकारेण समन्वितम्।

धारयेत्पञ्च घटिकाः वायुवद्व्योमगो भवेत्॥ २१॥

आकाशे वायुमारोप्य हकारोपरि शकरम्।

बिन्दुरूपं महादेवं व्योमाकारं सदाशिवम्॥ २२॥

शुद्धस्फटिकसङ्काशं बालेन्दुधृतमौलिनम्।

पञ्चवक्त्रयुतं सौम्यं दशबाहुं त्रिलोचनम्॥ २३॥

सर्वायुधोद्यतकरं सर्वाभरणभूषितम्।

उमार्धदेहं वरदं सर्वकारणकारणम्॥ २४॥

मनसा चिन्तयन्स्तु मुहूर्तमपि धारयेत्।

स एव मुक्त इत्युक्तस्तान्त्रिकेषु सुशिक्षितैः॥ २५॥

एतदुक्तं भवत्यत्र गार्गि ब्रह्मविदां वरे।

ब्रह्मादिकार्यरूपाणि स्वे स्वे संहृत्य कारणे॥ २६॥

तस्मिन्सदाशिवे प्राणं चित्तं चानीय कारणे।

युक्तचित्तस्तदात्मानं योजयेत्परमेश्वरे॥ २७॥

अस्मिन्नर्थे वदन्त्यन्ये योगिनो ब्रह्मविद्वराः।

प्रणवेनैव कार्याणि स्वे स्वे संहृत्य कारणे॥ २८॥

प्रणवस्य तु नादान्ते परमान्दविग्रहम्।

ऋतं सत्यं परं ब्रह्म पुरुषं कृष्णपिङ्गलम्॥ २९॥

चेतसा संप्रपश्यन्ति सन्तः संसारभेषजम्।

त्वं तस्मात् प्रणवेनैव प्राणायामैस्त्रिभिस्त्रिभिः॥ ३०॥

ब्रह्मादि कार्यरूपाणि स्वे स्वे संहृत्य कारणे।

विशुद्ध चेतसा पश्य नादान्ते परमेश्वरम्॥ ३१॥

अस्मिन्नर्थे वदन्त्यन्ये योगिनो ब्रह्मविद्वराः।

भिषग्वरा वरारोहे योगेषु परिनिष्ठिताः॥ ३२॥

शरीरं तावदेवं तु पञ्चभूतात्मकं खलु।

तदेतत्तु वरारोहे वातपित्तकफात्मकम्॥ ३३॥

वातात्मकानां सर्वेषां योगेष्वभिरतात्मनाम्।

प्राणसंयमनेनैव शोषं याति कलेवरम्॥ ३४॥

पित्तात्मकानां त्वचिरान्न शुष्यति कलेवरम्।

कफात्मकानां कायश्च सम्पूर्णस्त्वचिराद्भवेत्॥ ३५॥

धारणं कुर्वतस्त्वग्नौ सर्वे नश्यन्ति वातजाः।

पार्थिवांशे जलांशे च धारणं कुर्वतः सदा॥ ३६॥

नश्यन्ति श्लेष्मजा रोगा वातजाश्चाचिरात्तथा।

व्योमांशे मारुतांशे च धारणं कुर्वतः सदा॥ ३७॥

त्रिदोषजनिता रोगा विनश्यन्ति न संशयः।

अस्मिन्नर्थे तथाब्रूतामश्विनौ च भिषग्वराः॥ ३८॥

प्राणसंयमनेनैव त्रिदोषशमनं नृणाम्।

तस्मात्त्वं च वरारोहे नित्यं कर्म समाचर॥ ३९॥

यमादिभिश्च सम्युक्ता विधिवद्धारणं कुरु॥ ४०॥

इति श्रीयोगयाज्ञवल्क्ये अष्टमोऽध्यायः॥

नवमोऽध्यायः

याज्ञवल्क्य उवाच--

अथ ध्यानं प्रवक्ष्यामि श्रृणु गार्गि वरानने।

ध्यानमेव हि जन्तूनां कारणं बन्धमोक्षयोः ॥ १ ॥

ध्यानमात्मस्वरूपस्य वेदनं मनसा खलु।

सगुणं निर्गुणं तच्च सगुणं बहुशः स्मृतम् ॥ २ ॥

पञ्चोत्तमानि तेष्वाहुर्वैदिकानि द्विजोत्तमाः।

त्रीणि मुख्यतमान्येषामेकमेव हि निर्गुणं ॥ ३ ॥

मर्मस्थानानि नाडीनां संस्थानं च पृथक्पृथक्।

वायूनां स्थानकर्माणि ज्ञात्वा कुर्वात्मवेदनम् ॥ ४ ॥

एकं ज्योतिर्मयं शुद्धं सर्वगम् व्योमवत्क्रमम्।

अव्यक्तमचलं नित्यमादिमध्यान्तवर्जितम् ॥ ५ ॥

स्थूलम् सूक्ष्ममनाकारमसंस्पृश्यमचाक्षुषम्।

न रसं न च गन्धाख्यमप्रमेयमनौपमम् ॥ ६ ॥

आनन्दमजरं नित्यं सदसत्सर्वकारणम्।

सर्वाधारं जगद्रूपममूर्तमजमव्ययम् ॥ ७ ॥

अदृश्यं दृश्यमन्तःस्थं बहिःस्थं सर्वतोमुखम्।

सर्वदृक्सर्वतःपादं सर्वस्पृक् सर्वतःशिरः ॥ ८ ॥

ब्रह्म ब्रह्ममयोऽहं स्यामिति यद्वेदनं भवेत्।

तदेतन्निर्गुणं ध्यानमिति ब्रह्मविदो विदुः ॥ ९ ॥

अथवा परमात्मानं परमानन्दविग्रहम्।

गुरूपदेशाद्विज्ञाय पुरुषं कृष्णपिङ्गलम् ॥ १० ॥

ब्रह्म ब्रह्मपुरे चास्मिन्दहराम्बुजमध्यमे।

अभ्यासात्सम्प्रपश्यन्ति सन्तः संसारभेषजम् ॥ ११ ॥

हृत्पद्मेऽष्टदलोपेते कन्दमध्यात्समुत्थिते।

द्वादशाङ्गुलनालेऽस्मिंश्चतुरङ्गुलमुन्मुखे॥ १२॥

प्राणायामैर्विकासिते केसरान्वितकर्णिके।

वासुदेवं जगन्नाथं नारायणमजं हरिम्॥ १३॥

चतुर्भुजमुदाराङ्गं शङ्खचक्रगदाधरम्।

किरीटकेयूरधरं पद्मपत्रनिभेक्षणम्॥ १४॥

श्रीवत्सवक्षसं विष्णुं पूर्णचन्द्रनिभाननम्।

पद्मोदरदलाभोष्ठं सुप्रसन्नं शुचिस्मितम्॥ १५॥

शुद्धस्फटिकसङ्काशं पीतवाससमच्युतम्।

पद्मच्छविपदद्वन्द्वं परमात्मानमव्ययम्॥ १६॥

प्रभाभिर्भासयद्रूपं परितः पुरुषोत्तमम्।

मनसालोक्य देवेशं सर्वभूतहृदि स्थितम्॥ १७॥

सोऽहमात्मेति विज्ञानं सगुणं ध्यानमुच्यते।

हृत्सरोरुहमध्येऽस्मिन्प्रकृत्यात्मककर्णिके॥ १८॥

अष्टैश्वर्यदलोपेते विद्याकेसरसंयुते।

ज्ञाननाले बृहत्कन्दे प्राणायामप्रबोधिते॥ १९॥

विश्वार्चिषं महावह्निं ज्वलन्तं विश्वतोमुखम्।

वैश्वानरं जगद्योनिं शिखातन्विनमीश्वरम्॥ २०॥

तापयन्तं स्वकं देहमापादतलमस्तकम्।

निर्वातदीपवत्तस्मिन्दीपितं हव्यवाहनम्॥ २१॥

दृष्ट्वा तस्य शिखामध्ये परमात्मानमक्षरम्।

नीलतोयदमध्यस्थविद्युल्लेखेव भास्वरम्॥ २२॥

नीवारशूकवद्रूपं पीताभं सर्वकारणम्।

ज्ञात्वा वैश्वानरं देवं सोऽहमात्मेति या मतिः॥२३॥

सगुणेषूत्तमं ह्येतद्ध्यानं योगविदो विदुः।

वैश्वानरत्वं सम्प्राप्य मुक्तिं तेनैव गच्छति॥२४॥

अथवा मण्डले पश्येदादित्यस्य महाद्युतेः।

आत्मानं सर्वजगतः पुरुषं हेम रूपिणम्॥२५॥

हिरण्यश्मश्रुकेशं च हिरण्यमयनखं हरिम्।

कनकाम्बुजवद्वक्त्रं सृष्टिस्थित्यन्तकारणम्॥२६॥

पद्मासनस्थितं सौम्यं प्रबुद्धाब्जनिभाननम्।

पद्मोदरदलाभाक्षं सर्वलोकाभयप्रदम्॥२७॥

जानन्तं सर्वदा सर्वमुन्नयन्तं च धार्मिकान्।

भासयन्तं जगत्सर्वं दृष्ट्वा लोकैकसाक्षिणम्॥२८॥

सोऽहमस्मीति या बुद्धिः स च ध्यानेषु शस्यते।

एष एव तु मोक्षस्य महामार्गस्तपोधने॥२९॥

ध्यानेनानेन सौरेण मुक्तिं यास्यन्ति सूरयः।

भ्रुवोर्मध्येऽन्तरात्मानं भारूपं सर्वकारणम्॥३०॥

स्थाणुवन्मूर्धपर्यन्तं मध्यदेहात्मसमुत्थितम्।

जगत्कारणमव्यक्तं ज्वलन्तममितौजसम्॥३१॥

मनसालोक्य सोऽहं स्यामित्येतद्ध्यानमुत्तमम्।

अथवा बद्धपर्यङ्कं शितिलीकृतविग्रहे॥३२॥

शिव एव स्वयं भूत्वा नासाग्रारोपितेक्षणः।

निर्विकारं परं शान्तं परमात्मानमीश्वरं॥३३॥

भारूपममृतम् ध्यायेद्भ्रुवोर्मध्ये वरानने।

सोऽहमेवेति या बुद्धिः सा च ध्यानेषु शस्यते॥ ३४॥

अथवाष्टदलोपेते कर्णिकाकेसरान्विते।

उन्निद्रहृदयाम्भोजे सोममण्डलमध्यमे॥ ३५॥

स्वात्मानमर्भकाकारं भोक्तृरूपिणमव्ययम्।

सुधारसं विमुञ्चद्भिः शशिरश्मिभिरावृतम्॥ ३६॥

षोडशच्छदसंयुक्तशिरःपद्मादधोमुखात्।

निर्गतामृतधाराभिः सहस्राभिः समन्ततः॥ ३७॥

प्लावितं पुरुषं तत्र चिन्तयित्वा समाहितः।

तेनामृतरसेनैव साङ्गोपाङ्गकलेवरे॥ ३८॥

अहमेव परं ब्रह्म परमात्माहमव्ययः।

एवं यद्वेदनं तच्च सगुणं ध्यानमुच्यते॥ ३९॥

एवं ध्यानामृतम् कुर्वन् षन्मासान्मृत्युजिद्भवेत्।

वत्सरान्मुक्त एव स्याज्जीवन्नेव न संशयः॥ ४०॥

जीवन्मुक्तस्य न क्वापि दुःखावाप्तिः कथञ्चन।

किं पुनर्नित्यमुक्तस्य मुक्तिरेव हि दुर्लभा॥ ४१॥

तस्मात्त्वम् च वरारोहे फलम् त्यक्त्वैव नित्यशः।

विधिवत्कर्म कुर्वाणा ध्यानमेव सदा कुरु॥ ४२॥

अन्यानपि बहून्याहुर्ध्यानानि मुनिसत्तमाः।

मुख्यान्युक्तानि चैतेभ्यो जघन्यानीतराणि तु॥ ४३॥

सगुणं गुणहीनं वा विज्ञायात्मानमात्मनि।

सन्तः समाधिं कुर्वन्ति त्वमप्येवं सदा कुरु॥ ४४॥

इति श्रीयोगयाज्ञवल्क्ये नवमोऽध्यायः॥

दशमोऽध्यायः

याज्ञवल्क्य उवाच--

समाधिमधुना वक्ष्ये भवपाशविनाशनम्।

भवपाशनिबद्धस्य यथावच्छ्रोतुमर्हसि॥ १ ॥

समाधिः समतावस्था जीवात्मपरमात्मनोः।

ब्रह्मण्येव स्थितिर्या सा समाधिः प्रत्यगात्मनः॥ २ ॥

ध्यायेद्यथा यथात्मानं तत्समाधिस्तथा तथा।

ध्यात्वैवात्मनि संस्थाप्यो नान्यथात्मा यथा भवेत्॥ ३ ॥

एवमेव तु सर्वत्र यत्प्रपन्नस्तु यो नरः।

तदात्मा सोऽपि तत्रैव समाधिं समवाप्नुयात्॥ ४ ॥

सारित्पतौ निविष्टाम्बु यथाभिन्नतयान्वियात्।

तथात्माभिन्न एवात्र समाधिं समवाप्नुयात्॥ ५ ॥

एतदुक्तं भवत्यत्र गार्गि ब्रह्मविदां वरे।

कर्मैव विधिवत्कुर्वन्कामसङ्कल्पवर्जितम्॥ ६ ॥

वेदान्तेष्वथ शास्त्रेषु सुशिक्षितमनाः सदा।

गुरुणा तूपदिष्टार्थं युक्त्युपेतं वरानने॥ ७ ॥

विद्वद्भिर्धर्मशास्त्रज्ञैर्विचार्य च पुनः पुनः।

तस्मिन्सुनिश्चितार्थेषु सुशिक्षितमनाः सदा॥ ८ ॥

योगमेवाभ्यसेन्नित्यं जीवात्मपरमात्मनोः।

ततस्त्वाभ्यन्तरैश्चिह्नैर्बाह्यैर्वा कालसूचकैः॥ ९ ॥

विनिश्चित्यात्मनः कालमन्यैर्वा परमार्थवित्।

निर्भयः सुप्रसन्नात्मा मर्त्यस्तु विजितेन्द्रियः॥ १० ॥

स्वकर्मनिरतः शान्तः सर्वभूतहिते रतः।
प्रदाय विद्यां पुत्रस्य मन्त्रं च विधिपूर्वकम्॥ ११ ॥
संस्कारमात्मनः सर्वमुपदिश्य तदानघे।
पुण्यक्षेत्रे शुचौ देशे विद्वद्भिश्च समावृते॥ १२ ॥
भूमौ कुशान्समास्तीर्य कृष्णाजिनमथापि वा।
तस्मिन्सुबद्धपर्यङ्को मन्त्रैर्बद्धकलेवरः॥ १३ ॥
आसने नान्यधीरास्ते प्राङ्मुखो वाप्युदङ्मुखः।
नवद्वाराणि संयम्य गार्ग्यस्मिन्ब्रह्मणः पुरे॥ १४॥
उन्निद्रहृदयाम्भोजे प्राणायामैः प्रबोधिते।
व्योम्नि तस्मिन्प्रभारूपे स्वरूपे सर्वकारणे॥ १५॥
मनोवृत्तिं सुसंयम्य परमात्मनि पण्डितः।
मूर्ध्न्याधायात्मनः प्राणं भ्रुवोर्मध्येऽथवानघे॥ १६ ॥
कारणे परमानन्दे आस्थितो योगधारणाम्।
ओमित्येकाक्षरं बुद्ध्या व्याहरन्सुसमाहितः॥ १७॥
शरीरं संत्यजेद्विद्वानात्मैवाभून्नरोत्तमः।
यस्मिन्समभ्यसेद्विद्वान्योगेनैवात्मदर्शनम्॥ १८॥
तदेव सम्स्मरन्विद्वांस्त्यजेदन्ते कलेवरम्।
यं यं सम्यक्स्मरन्भावं त्यजत्यन्ते कलेवरम्॥ १९॥
तम् तमेवैत्यसौ भावमिति योगविदो विदुः।
त्वं चैवं योगमास्थाय ध्यायन्स्वात्मानमात्मनि॥ २०॥
स्वधर्मनिरता शान्ता त्यजान्ते देहमात्मनः।
ज्ञानेनैव सहैतेन नित्यकर्माणि कुर्वतः॥ २१॥

निवृत्तफलसङ्गस्य मुक्तिर्गार्गि करे स्थिता।

यदुक्तं ब्रह्मणा पूर्वं कर्मयोगसमुच्चयम्॥ २२॥

तदेतत्कीर्तितम् सर्वं साङ्गोपाङ्गं विधानतः।

त्वं चैव योगमभ्यस्य यमाद्यष्टाङ्गसम्युतम्॥ २३॥

निर्वाणं पदमासाद्य प्रपञ्चं संपरित्यज।

इति श्रीयोगयाज्ञवल्क्ये दशमोऽध्यायः॥

एकादशोऽध्यायः

इत्येवमुक्ता मुनिना याज्ञवल्क्येन धीमता।

ऋषिमध्ये वरारोहा वाक्यमेतदभाषत॥ १॥

गार्ग्युवाच--

योगयुक्तो नरः स्वामिन्सन्ध्ययोर्वाथवा सदा।

वैधं कर्म कथं कुर्यान्निष्कृतिः का त्वकुर्वतः॥ २॥

इत्युक्तो ब्रह्मवादिन्या ब्रह्मविद्ब्राह्मणस्तदा।

तां समालोक्य भगवानिदमाह नरोत्तमः॥ ३॥

याज्ञवल्क्य उवाच--

योगयुक्तमनुष्यस्य सन्ध्ययोर्वाथवा निशि।

यत्कर्तव्यं वरारोहे योगेन खलु तत्कृतम्॥ ४॥

आत्माग्निहोत्रवह्नौ तु प्राणायामैर्विवर्धिते।

विशुद्धचित्तहविषा विध्युक्तं कर्म जुह्वतः॥ ५॥

निष्कृतिस्तस्य किं बाले कृतकृत्यस्तदा खलु।

वियोगे सति सम्प्राप्ते जीवात्मपरमात्मनोः॥ ६॥

विध्युक्तं कर्म कर्तव्यं ब्रह्मविद्भिश्च नित्यशः।

वियोगकाले योगी च दुःखमित्येव यस्त्यजेत्॥७॥

कर्माणि तस्य निलयः निरयः परिकीर्तितः।

न देहिनां यतः शक्यं त्यक्तुं कर्माण्यशेषतः॥८॥

तस्मादामरणाद्वैधं कर्तव्यं योगिभिः सदा।

त्वं चैव मात्यया गार्गि वैधं कर्म समाचर॥९॥

योगेन परमात्मानं यजंस्त्यज कलेवरम्।

इत्येवमुक्त्वा भगवान्याज्ञवल्क्यस्तपोनिधिः॥१०॥

ऋशीनालोक्य नेत्राभ्यां वाक्यमेतदभाषत।

सन्ध्यामुपास्य विधिवत्पश्चिमां सुसमाहिताः॥११॥

गच्छन्तु साम्प्रतं सर्वे ऋषयः स्वाश्रमं प्रति।

इत्येवमुक्ता मुनिना मुनयः संश्रितव्रताः॥१२॥

विश्वामित्रो वसिष्ठश्च गौतमश्चाङ्गिरास्तथा।

अगस्त्यो नारदश्चैव वाल्मीकिर्बादरायणिः॥१३॥

पैङ्गिदीर्घतमा व्यासः शौनकश्च तपोधनः।

भार्गवः काश्यपश्चैव भरद्वाजस्तथैव च॥१४॥

तपस्विनस्तथा चान्ये वेदवेदाङ्गवेदिनः।

याज्ञवल्क्यं सुसम्पूज्य गीर्भिराशीर्भिरुत्तमैः॥१५॥

ते यान्ति मुनयः सर्वे स्वाश्रमेषु यथागतम्।

गतेषु स्वाश्रमेष्वेषु तापसेषु तपोधना॥१६॥

प्रणम्य दण्डवद्भूमौ वाक्यमेतदभाषत।

गार्ग्युवाच--

भगवन्सर्वशास्त्रज्ञ सर्वभूतहिते रत॥१७॥

भवमोक्षाय योगीन्द्र भवद्भिर्भाषितम् तु यत्।

यमाद्यष्टाङ्गसहितो योगो मुक्तेस्तु साधनम्॥ १८॥

तदेतद्विस्मृतम् सर्वं सर्वज्ञं तव सन्निधौ।

योगं ममोपदिश्याद्य साङ्गं सङ्क्षेपरूपतः॥ १९॥

त्रातुमर्हसि सर्वज्ञ जन्मसंसारसागरात्।

इत्युक्तो ब्रह्मवादिन्या ब्रह्मविद्ब्राह्मणस्तदा॥ २०॥

आलोक्य कृपया दीनां स्मितपूर्वमभाषत।

उत्तिष्ठोत्तिष्ठ किं शेषे भूमौ गार्गि वरानने॥ २१॥

वक्ष्यामि ते समासेन योगं सम्प्रति तं शृणु॥

इति श्रीयोगयाज्ञवल्क्ये एकादशोऽध्यायः॥

द्वादशोऽध्यायः

सव्येन गुल्फेन गुदम् निपीड्य सव्येतरेणैव निपीड्य सन्धिम्॥

सव्येतरं न्यस्य करेतरस्मिन्शिखां समालोकय पावकस्य॥ १॥

आयुर्विधातकृत्प्राणो निरुद्धस्त्वासनेन वै।

याति गार्गि तदापानत् कुलं वह्नेः शनैः शनैः॥ २॥

वायुना वातितो वह्निरपानेन शनैः शनैः।

ततो ज्वलति सर्वेषां स्वकुले देहमध्यमे॥ ३॥

प्रातःकाले प्रदोषे च निशीथे च समाहितः।

मुहूर्तमभ्यसेदेवम् यावत् पञ्चदिनद्वयम्॥ ४॥

ततस्त्वात्मनि विप्रेन्द्रे प्रत्ययाश्च पृथक्पृथक्।

सम्भवन्ति तदा तस्य जितो येन समीरणः॥ ५॥

शरीरलघुता दीप्तिर्वह्नेर्जठरवर्तिनः।

नादाभिव्यक्तिरित्येते चिह्नान्यादौ भवन्ति हि॥ ६॥
अल्पमूत्रपुरीषः स्यात्षण्मासे वत्सरेऽपि वा।
आसने वाहने पश्चान्न भेतव्यं त्रिवत्सरात्॥ ७॥
ततोऽनिलं वायुसखेन सार्धं धिया समारोप्य निरोधयेत्तम्।
ध्यायन्सदा चक्रिणमप्रबुद्धम् नाभौ सदा कुण्डलिनीनिविष्टम्॥ ८॥
शिरां समावेष्य मुखेन मध्यामन्याश्च भोगेन शिरास्तथैव।
स्वपुच्छमास्येन निगृह्य सम्यक्पथश्च संयम्य मरुद्गणानाम्॥ ९॥
प्रसुप्तनागेन्द्रवदुच्छ्वसन्ती सदा प्रबुद्धा प्रभया ज्वलन्ती।
नाभौ सदा तिष्ठति कुन्डली सा तिर्यक्सु देहेषु तथेतरेषु॥ १०॥
वायुना विहतवह्निशिखाभिः कन्दमध्यगतनाडीषु संस्थाम्।
कुण्डलीं दहति यस्त्वहिरूपाम् संस्मरन्नरवरस्तु स एव॥ ११॥
सन्तप्ता वह्निना तत्र वायुना च प्रचालिता।
प्रसार्य फणभृद्भोगं प्रबोधम् याति सा तदा॥ १२॥
बोधं गते चक्रिणि नाभिमध्ये प्राणाः सुसम्भूय कलेवरेऽस्मिन्।
चरन्ति सर्वे सह वह्निनैव यथा पटे तन्तुगतिस्तथैव॥ १३॥
जित्वैवम् चक्रिणः स्थानं सदा ध्यानपरायणः।
ततो नयेदपानं तो नाभेरूर्ध्वमिदं स्मरन्॥ १४॥
वायुर्यथा वायुसखेन सार्धं नाभिं त्वतिक्रम्य गतः शरीरे।
रोगाश्च नश्यन्ति बलाभिवृद्धिः कान्तिस्तदानीमभवत्प्रबुद्धे॥ १५॥
ब्रह्मरन्ध्रमुखमत्र वायवः पावकेन सह यान्ति समूह्य।
केनचिदिह वदामि तवाहं वीक्षणाद् हृदि सुदीपशिखायाः॥ १६॥
निरोधितः स्याद्धृदि तेन वायुः मध्ये यदा वायुसखेन सार्धम्।

सहस्रपत्रस्य मुखं प्रविश्य कुर्यात्पुनस्तूर्ध्वमुखं द्विजेन्द्रे॥ १७॥

प्रबुद्धहृदयाम्भोजे गार्ग्यस्मिन्ब्रह्मणः पुरे।

बालार्कश्रेणिवद्व्योम्नि विरराज समीरणः॥ १८॥

हृन्मध्यात्तु सुषुम्नायां संस्थितो हुतभुक्तदा।

सजलाम्बुदमालासु विद्युल्लेखेव राजते॥ १९॥

प्रबुद्धहृत्पद्मनि संस्थितेऽग्नौ प्राणे च तस्मिन्विनिवेशिते च।

चिह्नानि बाह्यानि तथान्तराणि दीपादि दृश्याणि भवन्ति तस्य॥ २०॥

वायुमुन्नय ततस्तु सवह्निं व्याहरन्प्रणवमत्र सबिन्दुं।

बालचन्द्रसदृशे तु ललाटे बालचन्द्रमवलोकय बुद्ध्या॥ २१॥

सवह्निं वायुमारोप्य भ्रुवोर्मध्ये धिया तदा।

ध्यायेदनन्यधीः पश्चादन्तरात्मानमन्तरे॥ २२॥

मध्यमेऽपि हृदये च ललाटे स्थाणुवज्ज्वलति लिङ्गमदृश्यम्।

अस्ति गार्गि परमार्थमिदं त्वं पश्य पश्य मनसा रुचिरूपम्॥ २३॥

ललाटमध्ये हृदयाम्बुजे च यः पश्यति ज्ञामयीं प्रभां तु।

शक्तिं सदा दीपवदुज्ज्वलन्तीं स पश्यति ब्रह्मविदेकादृष्ट्या॥ २४॥

मनो लयम् यदा याति भ्रूमध्ये योगिनाम् नृणाम्।

जिह्वामूलेऽमृतस्रावो भ्रूमध्ये चात्मदर्शनम्॥ २५॥

कम्पनं च तथा मूर्ध्नो मनसैवात्मदर्शनं।

देवोद्यानानि रम्याणि नक्षत्राणि च चन्द्रमाः॥

ऋषयः सिद्धगन्धर्वाः प्रकाशं यान्ति योगिनाम्॥ २६॥

भ्रुवोन्तरे विष्णुपदे ऋचौ तु मनो लयम् यावदियात्प्रबुद्धे।

तावत्समभ्यस्य पुनः खमध्ये सुखम् सदा संस्मर पूर्णरूपम्॥ २७॥

समीरणे विष्णुपदे निविष्टे जीवे च तस्मिन्नमृते च संस्थे।
तस्मिन्स्तदा याति मनो लयं चेन्मुक्तेः समीपं तदिति ब्रुवन्ति॥ २८॥
समीरणे विष्णुपदे निविष्टे विशुद्धबुद्धौ च तदात्मनिष्ठे।
आनन्दमत्यद्भुतमस्ति सत्यं त्वं गार्गि पश्याद्य विशुद्धबुद्ध्या॥ २९॥
एवं समभ्यस्य सुदीर्घकालं यमादिभिर्युक्ततनुर्मिताशीः।
आत्मानमासाद्य गुहां प्रविष्टं मुक्तिं व्रज ब्रह्मपुरे पुनस्त्वम्॥ ३०॥
भूतानि यस्मात्प्रभवन्ति गार्गि येनैव जीवन्ति चराचराणि।
जातानि यस्मिन्विलयं प्रयान्ति तद्ब्रह्म विद्धीति वदन्ति सर्वे॥ ३१॥
हृत्पङ्कजे व्योम्नि यदेकरूपं सत्यं सदानन्दमयं सुसूक्ष्मम्।
तद्ब्रह्म निर्भासमयं गुहायामिति श्रुतिश्चेति समामनन्ति॥ ३२॥
अणोरणीयान्महतो महीयानात्मा गुहायं निहितोऽस्य जन्तोः।
तमक्रतुं पश्य विशुद्धबुद्ध्या प्रयाणकाले च विहीनशोका॥ ३३॥
प्रभञ्जनं मूर्ध्निगतं सवह्निं धिया समासाद्य गुरूपदेशात्।
मूर्धानमुद्भिद्य पुनः खमध्ये प्राणास्त्यजोङ्कारमनुस्मरंस्त्वम्॥ ३४॥
ईप्सया यदि शरीरविसर्गं ज्ञातुमिच्चसि सखे तव वक्ष्ये।
व्याहरन्प्रणवमुन्नय मूर्ध्नि भिद्य योजय तमात्मनिकायम्॥ ३५॥
एतत्पवित्रं परमं योगमष्टाङ्गसंयुतम्।
ज्ञानं गुह्यतमं पुण्यं कीर्तितं ते वरानने॥ ३६॥
य इदम् श्र्णुयान्नित्यं योगाख्यानं नरोत्तमः।
सर्वपापविनिर्मुक्तः सम्यग्ज्ञानी भविष्यति॥ ३७॥
यस्त्वेतच्छ्रावयेद्विद्वान्नित्यं भक्तिसमन्वितः।
एकजन्मकृतं पापं दिनेनैकेन नश्यति॥ ३८॥

श्रृणुयाद्यः सकृद्वापि योगाख्यानमिदं नरः।

अज्ञानजनितं पापं सर्वं तस्य प्रणश्यति॥ ३९॥

अनुतिष्ठन्ति ये नित्यमात्मज्ञानसमन्वितम्।

नित्यकर्माणि तान्दृष्ट्वा देवाश्च प्रणमन्ति हि॥ ४०॥

तस्माज्ज्ञानेन देहान्तं नित्यं कर्म यथावधि।

कर्तव्यं देहिभिर्गार्गि योगश्च भवभीरुभिः॥ ४१॥

इत्येवमुक्त्वा भगवान्रहस्ये रहस्यजं मुक्तिकरं तु तुस्याः।

योगामृतं बन्धविनाशहेतुं समाधिमास्ते रहसि द्विजेन्द्रः॥ ४२॥

स तं तु सम्पूज्य मुनिं ब्रुवन्तं विद्यानिधिं ब्रह्मविदां वरिष्ठम्।

गीर्भिः प्रणामैश्च सतां वरिष्ठं सदा मुदम् प्राप वरां विशुद्धाम्॥ ४३॥

योगं सुसङ्गृह्य तदा रहस्ये रहस्यजं मुक्तिकरं च जन्तोः।

सम्सारमुत्सृज्य सदा मुदान्विता वने रहस्यावसथे विवेश॥ ४४॥

येन प्रपञ्चं परिपूर्णमेतद्येनैव विश्वं प्रतिभाति सर्वम्।

तं वासुदेवं श्रुतिमूर्ध्नि जातं पश्यन्सदास्ते हृदि मूर्ध्नि चान्वहम्॥ ४५॥

यदेकमव्यक्तमनन्तमच्युतं प्रपञ्चजन्मादिकृदप्रमेयम्।

तं वासुदेवं श्रुतिमूर्ध्नि जातं पश्यन्सदास्ते हृदि मूर्ध्नि चान्वहम्॥ ४६॥

इति श्रीयोगयाज्ञवल्क्ये द्वादशोऽध्यायः॥

समाप्तमिदं योगशास्त्रम्॥

About the Translators

The word *Svastha* in Sanskrit refers to the state of complete health and balance. Svastha Yoga & Ayurveda was founded by A. G. Mohan and Indra Mohan.

A. G. Mohan was a personal student of Sri T. Krishnamacharya from 1971 to 1989. He was also the convener of Krishnamacharya's centenary celebrations in 1988. He is the author of *Yoga for Body, Breath, and Mind* (1993) with a foreword from Krishnamacharya himself, *Yoga Therapy* (2004), and *Krishnamacharya: His Life and Teachings* (2010).

Indra Mohan has been practicing and teaching yoga for more than three decades now. She is one of the few people who received a post-graduate diploma in yoga from Krishnamacharya.

Ganesh Mohan, son of A. G. Mohan and Indra Mohan, was trained from childhood in yoga and other related areas such as Vedic chanting. He is a doctor, formally trained in both modern medicine and ayurveda. He is the co-author of the Mohans' books, *Yoga Therapy* and *Krishnamacharya.* He is deeply interested in the profound wisdom of the Yogasūtra of Patañjali, which he continues to study and teach.

Nitya Mohan, daughter of A. G. Mohan and Indra Mohan, was trained in yoga from a young age. She holds a degree in music and is an exponent of Vedic chanting. She runs the Svastha training program in Singapore and has released audio recordings on Vedic chanting and the Yogasūtra of Patañjali.

Made in the USA
Las Vegas, NV
03 April 2023

70124117R00105